A CHANGE FOR THE BETTER

A CHANGE FOR THE BETTER

*How to survive – and thrive –
during the menopause*

Dr Hilary Jones

Hodder & Stoughton

First published in Great Britain in 2000 by Hodder and Stoughton
A division of Hodder Headline

10 9 8 7 6 5 4

A CIP catalogue record for this title is available from the British Library.

ISBN 0 340 76810 X

Diagrams by Rodney Paull

Typeset in Palatino by
Phoenix Typesetting, Ilkley, West Yorkshire

Printed and bound in Great Britain by
Mackays of Chatham plc, Chatham, Kent

Hodder and Stoughton
A division of Hodder Headline
338 Euston Road
London NW1 3BH

To Evan and Noreen
and to all the women who are simply not prepared
to allow the menopause to get in the way of the
rest of their lives

ACKNOWLEDGEMENTS

I should like to thank all those people who have contributed so actively towards the research necessary for the compilation of this book. In particular I should like to thank Bonnie Green and her colleagues at Henderson Group One, Dr Val Godfree of the Amarant Trust, Linda Edwards, director of the National Osteoporosis Society and Toni Belfield and her colleagues at the Family Planning Association. I am also indebted to Joan Jenkins OBE, who founded the Women's Health Concern Movement in 1972, and inspired by her continued enthusiasm and dedication to propagating accurate and helpful messages regarding hormone replacement therapy. If her energy and drive has anything to do with the fact that she herself has been taking HRT for over 28 years and continues to do so, I think I may be tempted to start taking it myself!

I must thank Dr Graham E. Kelly who provided me with such excellent state-of-the-art research material on the subject of phytoestrogens and Dr Maryon Stewart of the Women's Nutritional Advisory Service for her input into nutritional therapy for the menopause generally. Also, I am very grateful to Charles Worthington, British Hairdresser of the Year, for his valuable input.

Finally, a huge thank you to my wife Sarah and our good friend Jane Ledger for their painstaking and laborious attention to detail in compiling, typing and editing the manuscript. Without them, the book could never have come to fruition.

CONTENTS

AUTHOR'S NOTE

This book is intended as a guide to women who want to improve their health during the menopause. If you are concerned in any way about your health, you should seek specific medical advice from your own family practitioner.

Advances, alterations and refinements in modern therapeutics mean that some of the information contained in this book regarding HRT and other treatment for the menopause may soon become out of date. This is particularly relevant to the pharmaceutical information found in Chapter 14, although all information was correct at the time of going to print.

FOREWORD

I think this book, with its refreshingly upbeat title, 'A Change for the Better', should be compulsory reading for any woman of any age who wants to know more about the menopause. When you think that women, who make up half the world's population, will at some stage experience some of the symptoms of the menopause and that the majority will still suffer in silence from the physical and psychological problems that hormone changes may bring, it is easy to see just how important this book will be.

My own mother went through a dreadful time when she had her menopause, with terrible hot flushes and incredibly heavy and irregular periods, and as her daughter I was very concerned about her at the time and desperately wished she could have had more help and support. They say that daughters often go through a menopause at about the same age and with the same severity of symptoms as their mother did, so I read *A Change for the Better* with particular interest and I know I will find it invaluable again later when my ovaries stop talking to me. No menopausal woman should have to suffer as my mother did, and with the help of this book, no one need to do so in the future.

It's packed with easy to understand information and really practical tips and recommendations about how to avoid problems to begin with. For the first time I now actually understand why the menopause happens and feel I will be able in the future to make a clear and sensible decision about HRT or any of the natural and complementary alternatives.

The Menopause Assessment Scale in Chapter 6 is especially useful in helping you to gauge the severity of any symptoms you may have and what you should do about them, and the section on phytoestrogens – the oestrogens which are derived from plants – is both fascinating and very well researched.

The truth about HRT can be found here too. As a TV presenter

I am so aware of the confusion and polarisation of views about whether or not to take HRT. Here at last is a book that tells us everything we ever wanted to know about HRT, set up in a clear, logical and unbiased fashion. But knowing Dr Hilary Jones as I do from the GMTV sofa, I would not expect anything less. When it comes to obtaining information and advice about health we need to trust our doctors and advisors absolutely, and with Hilary, you just know you're getting advice you can totally rely on.

The menopause need not be a hurdle in any woman's life at all. In fact there are many definite benefits which may be associated with new-found freedoms and independence. It simply isn't true that your family and society as a whole will regard you as socially redundant after the menopause, nor is it the case that your appearance or your love life should suffer.

So if you, or someone you know, is being held back in any way by the experience of the menopause, this is the book you need. It will foster a positive and healthy approach to the menopause, which with very little effort can definitely become 'A Change for the Better'.

Fiona
Phillips

INTRODUCTION

Every woman can expect to experience the menopause one day. But each individual woman's own experience will be unique and totally different. Perhaps that is just one of the reasons why, with so many words published and broadcast on the subject, so much confusion and misunderstanding about the menopause and its management still abounds.

In Britain today, most women will spend more than one third of their entire life post-menopausally, so it is vitally important that should they be one of the unlucky ones who develop moderate or severe symptoms, they should not simply be prepared to grin and bear it and to suffer in silence as their mothers and grandmothers before them certainly did.

Tragically, however, I know many women still do suffer terribly. In my own surgery over the years I have seen many patients who I have known as strong, stoical, well-informed and capable women who have been devastated by the effects of a bad menopause. Some have not even recognised the underlying problem. One, I remember, felt she was losing her mind. She felt guilty about constantly snapping at her teenage children, frightened that her partner would leave her because of her lack of interest in sex , and tearful and depressed about her weight gain and inability to sleep at night. It would have been the easiest thing in the world to provide her with an antidepressant, yet it would have been a mistake. She was basically menopausal and experiencing predominantly psychological symptoms resulting from measurable oestrogen deficiency. Simple tests proved this and she responded dramatically to hormone replacement. Had she been prescribed antidepressants they would have done nothing to alleviate any symptoms other than depression and might well have resulted in unnecessary and unpleasant side effects.

Another patient merely asked me for advice. She had next to no menopausal symptoms whatsoever but wondered whether such a happy scenario was actually normal.

A third woman had heard that HRT would dramatically enhance her love life. A famous celebrity actress had publicly boasted about the four toyboy lovers she had taken since she had started taking HRT. I had to explain tactfully that that level of expectation was unfortunately likely to lead to disappointment.

Clearly, if ever you had a call for an holistic approach to a common and important physiological event encompassing your physical, psychological *and* emotional needs, the menopause is a great example.

There were several reasons why I wanted to write this book. First, the menopause affects almost everyone. Women make up just over half of the entire population yet their partners and their children may also be touched by the consequences of menopausal symptoms too. Secondly, it has been a badly neglected area of medicine historically. Negative attitudes are only now beginning to change. Thirdly, there are numerous myths which need exploding and much public confusion which needs addressing. Many doctors openly admit they are not up to date with the latest advances in contemporary hormone replacement therapy nor the numerous alternatives to HRT which are now on offer. Some doctors feel the menopause is unworthy of treatment, full stop. The polarisation of views concerning HRT amongst members of the public is truly alarming. Whilst some women proclaim it as the best thing since sliced bread, others decry it as an unnecessary poison, an instrument of the devil dished out by doctors who have been bribed to prescribe it by a conniving and predominantly greed-motivated pharmaceutical industry. On GMTV recently I argued against a highly publicised opponent of HRT who not only held this very opinion but also claimed she knew of several women who had grown penises whilst taking HRT. As I countered that this was plainly ridiculous and that the lady in question should never have been offered air-time, the regular breakfast TV presenters dissolved into uncontrollable laughter and almost fell off the famous studio sofa! Some viewers were shocked. Many phoned in to say that my adversary had caused more harm to the anti-HRT movement than any other single person in the last ten years. Others who had been more than happy on HRT were needlessly alarmed and may well have become very anxious about alleged side effects or the suggestion that their long-term health might somehow be at risk.

This is the kind of background which motivated me to write this book. There were also all sorts of exciting developments in the field of dietary manipulation, for example discoveries about the value of plant-derived oestrogens (phytoestrogens) and how incorporating them into a regular eating plan could ease menopausal symptoms. Pharmaceutical companies are now exploring synthetic modifications of such hormones with a view to providing ever-increasingly effective treatment for oestrogen-dependent cancers in the future.

But I make no apology for the fact that a book designed almost exclusively for women – to empower them to face up to the menopause and its challenges – is penned by a male author, even if his Christian name is Hilary! I cannot speak about the menopause from personal experience of course, but then I do not know what it is like to have a brain tumour, meningitis or kidney stones either. That does not mean I cannot empathise, reach out to patients and be a caring and effective therapist. Most gynaecologists are, in fact, men. Yet gynaecologists of either sex cannot discern any obvious professional advantage when it comes to matters of gender. And just as many female doctors are accused of being unsympathetic and dismissive of patients as male doctors are of being out of touch and condescending. I have tried very hard to remain aware of gender discriminations and, hopefully, I have compensated accordingly.

In this new millennium the menopause need no longer be regarded by women as a time they must come to dread. It need no longer be associated as it once was with negative attitudes, intractable physical symptoms and mind-altering psychological turmoil. Nor should it any longer be the subject of such widespread but misguided medical mythology. HRT does *not* make you gain weight. You do not suddenly cease to be sexually attractive or responsive, you do not become socially redundant in the eyes of your family and society as a whole and it is not the final chapter in a woman's intellectual life by any means. Far from it. We now have wonderfully beneficial ways of solving difficulties when and if they arise. The future for women experiencing the menopause is very bright. So whether women rely on simple self-help measures, natural oestrogens in their diet, a variety of complementary medicines or the latest formulations of hormone replacement therapy, their 'change' as it is still commonly called, can now become 'a change for the better'.

PART ONE

CHAPTER ONE

A CHANGE FOR THE BETTER

Different Attitudes Towards the Menopause

Every woman's experience of and attitude to the menopause is individual and unique. Regrettably, in contemporary Western society, the majority of women still see the menopause as a time of unwelcome and distressing change in psychological and spiritual as well as physical ways. This widespread and unnecessary stereotypical attitude towards the menopause is unhelpful because it can bring with it a damaging form of victim mentality from which the woman experiencing it can find it difficult to escape. Such a negative outlook undoubtedly has a major bearing on how you might adapt to your menopause and how you tolerate any symptoms that you have. It is sad that the menopause has such a bad press and that women are so often bombarded with horror stories about it. Considering that in many ways we all create our own reality, the more we expect bad things to happen, the more likely they are to do so. Instead of thinking so negatively it is worth remembering that the menopause can bring very positive and rewarding benefits if you are able to focus on these and be encouraged to view the situation differently. It is only in the Western world that such a negative approach to the menopause has been allowed to gain momentum, and I firmly believe that, given the right support, the correct information and a balanced view, the vast majority of women can come to look upon the menopause not as a time in their life to dread and endure but a time to look forward to a refreshing and constructive adjustment of their role within society, with their new-found freedom from grown-up children and their welcome and long over-due independence. In short, they can come to believe with absolute conviction that the change they are experiencing is a positive and welcome change and one in fact which is very much a change for the better.

As a GP, I am constantly amazed by how differently different women perceive the significance of the menopause. In my consultation room some women are obviously agitated and depressed about what is happening to them, and the disintegration of their self-esteem and well-being is clear for all to see. By contrast others come in to announce that they are using their new-found freedom to travel the world or set up a new business. And of course many never mention their menopausal symptoms at all, believing that the changes they notice, if any, are not symptoms of a medical disorder as such and therefore not within the usual remit of a medical consultation.

These conflicting attitudes are reflected in equal measure by the post bag I receive as a medical broadcaster in television and radio. Some women appear to be shocked and psychologically paralysed by the onset of their menopausal symptoms, whereas others have adjusted quickly to their new roles in life and their independence and are using their new-found energy and enthusiasm to campaign on behalf of others in their work for charities or other self-help organisations and are branching out into all kinds of novel and interesting activities. Perhaps this range of differing outlooks towards the menopause can be neatly summed up by the experiences of three women, namely Rosemary, Christine and Kelly.

Rosemary looked tired and complained of overwhelming exhaustion. In the last few months she had been sleeping very badly, often finding it difficult to get to sleep to begin with and then waking up in the middle of the night with her nightie soaked through with sweat. She would climb out of bed and throw open the windows, much to the disgust of her husband who had already been telling her that she had become grumpy, irritable and difficult to live with. Rosemary would then take an hour or two to get back to sleep and consequently felt very aware of her fatigue and lack of alertness the following day. She had recently begun to experience embarrassing episodes of sweating, reporting a wave of heat that would begin around her face and neck and then spread downwards to engulf her whole body in an obvious rash. These hot flushes would generally last only a minute or two, but they were always severe enough to cause her to lose concentration at work and make it impossible for her to stay in the kitchen and prepare the evening meal or to sit in the confines of the stuffy coffee room at work. In the last fortnight she had started to avoid activities she had always been extremely keen on such as her yoga class, the opera or even shopping at the supermarket since she had begun to feel claustrophobic, uncertain and prone to be panicky in such circumstances. Rosemary privately had begun to feel that she had become sexually unattractive, that she was overweight, looked terrible and was now totally over the hill. She believed that her husband's criticism reflected his growing contempt of her and sometimes, on the worst days, that her life was almost not worth living. She had contemplated going to see her doctor about hormone replacement therapy but considered, rightly or wrongly, that HRT was really for women with plenty of 'go' and who craved a rampant libido. She had avoided making an appointment as she felt her doctor would also be unlikely to take much of an interest in her, especially in view of the way she currently felt about herself.

Christine had noticed some minor irregularities in her periods when she was 49, at roughly the same time that she met John with whom she began a relationship. For the first time in many years she felt cherished and cared for, and she and John embarked upon an extended holiday to Australasia then set up a business together. She felt so fulfilled and happy that she barely noticed that her periods had stopped altogether, and 15 months after her last period she went to the family planning clinic to check whether she needed to continue with contraception or not. She was sexually active and totally fulfilled in that aspect of her life, and she was thrilled by the challenge and excitement of her new career in making and selling pottery.

When Kelly attended the surgery for the third time in two weeks, she was crying. She felt guilty that she was unable to function and desperately worried that the rest of her family thought badly of her inability to cope with her problems. She felt that she was going completely mad at times, she could not concentrate, she was moody and irritable and had been totally uninterested in any of the romantic advances that her husband had made to her for many more months than she could remember. Her muscles and joints ached all over, her hair was thin and her skin coarse and dry; she was plagued by hot flushes and night sweats. She suffered constant vaginal irritation and had had a number of urinary infections of late which were inconvenient and made her anxious. Her sleeping pattern was disastrous, resulting in increasing day-time fatigue which only made her depression worse. Kelly was experiencing very severe symptoms of the menopause being amongst the unlucky 20 per cent of women who do, and her attendance at the surgery was the first correct step she had taken in order to find an effective solution.

These three women's experiences of the menopause, their symptoms and their attitudes bear testimony to the fact that every woman's journey through 'the change' is different and exclusive to her. Symptoms, if they arise at all, can always be treated in one way or another. Negative feelings and despondency, however, can only be corrected over a period of time, and preferably with the help of changing attitudes in society. If we look more deeply we can see how the stereotypical negative attitude towards the menopause may have come about.

The Perceived Horror of the Menopause

At least three-quarters of all women in the Western world will notice a number of rapid changes and unwanted symptoms during their menopause. These will often be sufficient to disrupt their normal life and cause a significant degree of inconvenience and misery. Amongst the commonest symptoms are hot flushes and night sweats, closely followed by fatigue, disorientation and depression. At the same time many women experience vaginal dryness and sometimes pain during love-making leading to a reduction in libido and avoidance of sex. Insomnia, lack of concentration and irritability are often reported. Media coverage of all these physical symptoms and psychological manifestations encourages most women to believe that the menopause is a horrendous period of their lives which will be most uncomfortable and will bring changes in the way other people regard them. Most women realise that the menopause is related to a state of oestrogen deficiency which in itself conjures up images of something being lacking, of inadequacy.

The role of oestrogen has in fact only fairly recently been properly understood, its original identification occurring late in the 1920s. At the beginning of the new millennium its application as a component of the oral contraceptive pill and of hormone replacement therapy now gives it its place in popular folklore as the hormone synonymous with femininity, sexuality and womanhood. Most women are aware that oestrogen is essential for the formation and function of the reproductive organs, in controlling the menstrual cycle, in pregnancy, in protecting women against heart disease and osteoporosis and in maintaining the physical integrity of healthy skin, attractive hair and strong beautiful nails. In contrast the menopausal state of oestrogen deficiency is portrayed as something that is dangerous to a woman's body and mind, and since these days women live, on average, well into their eighties, the fact that they spend over a third of their lives in a post-menopausal state makes many women wonder why nature has made the mistake of creating the menopause at all, and what purpose it could have had in evolutionary terms. Such negative thinking encourages women to believe that the menopause is the beginning of the descent into grey-haired old age when they will quickly become redundant as a lover and mother and that life will take a generally downhill path from this point.

Whilst many women feel a certain sadness and frustration with the onset of the menopause, society in general contributes to this feeling by associating physical ageing with loss of sexual attractiveness and self-esteem. Men feel this too when they are made acutely aware of a receding hair line, of a pot belly or even merely of a loss of rapport with younger people in the work place. In the home situation and amongst the family some women sense a loss of personal identity and a change in their role which is beyond their control. Others who have achieved much in their chosen careers discover a feeling that suddenly something is missing in their life and that part of it has passed them by.

Unfortunately, over the last 20 years our society's cultural attitudes about the menopause have merely served to reinforce these damaging perceptions. Oestrogen deficiency is not in itself a disease, and by no means do all women have to struggle through a menopause experiencing pain or grief. Certainly if women believe that they will, they are more likely to do so, and being encouraged to believe that they need treatment just as they need a new outfit, a new hairdo or even a new car does not help. There are plenty of other 'deficiency' disorders such as diabetes, where insulin is deficient, or Addison's Disease, where cortisol is deficient; and hormone replacement treatment for those life-threatening conditions is essential. But not all menopausal women whose oestrogen levels are waning need HRT, and to be made to feel inadequate simply because of not taking HRT is an unhealthy view.

Different Attitudes Towards the Menopause

I have encountered numerous different attitudes to the menopause amongst both health professionals and the general public. The traditional medical view of the menopause is that it is an unnatural state brought about by increased longevity. All other animals breed until they die; it is only because women no longer die from childhood diseases or through giving birth, and are living so many years longer than nature intended them to, that menopausal symptoms have become a modern problem. The argument goes that it is because women on the whole live an extra 30 or 40 years beyond the menopause that HRT has become necessary. The majority of doctors advise that treatment for the menopause both provides relief of unpleasant symptoms and prevents serious long-term complications such as brittle bone disease and heart disease.

These traditionalists of course have a point, but there is no doubt that the menopause and ageing generally have become unnecessarily 'medicalised' in all sorts of ways. There remains an over-eagerness to prescribe drugs and other therapies whilst ignoring the cultural and psychological effects. Almost all doctors are ready to prescribe HRT for high risk groups of women, although two-thirds are unhappy providing it for every woman over the age of 45, and a few remain totally opposed to HRT full stop. Even complementary practitioners have largely adopted the medical model of the menopause and have adapted their treatments and therapies accordingly, reinforcing at the same time the negative stereotype that is reflected in society.

Many people regard attitudes within society as being important determinants of how women see themselves and how they should react to the menopause. They have noticed how many other issues have become medicalised – the resistance to home deliveries in favour of childbirth in hospitals, and the psychiatric treatment of eating disorders which many regard as purely a feminist issue, being examples. They are equally angry that so many post-menopausal women are regarded as sexually and socially obsolete, and medically and emotionally out of control. They are critical of what they see as efforts by giant pharmaceutical companies to put HRT in the tap water as it were and provide it for all and sundry at great profit to themselves. They are frustrated with a society which values so highly the image of the young slim sexually attractive fashion model and allows cruel lampoons of the standard menopausal stereotype as characterised by caricature creations of comedians such as Les Dawson, the Monty Python team or even female comediennes such as Dawn French and Jennifer Saunders. More worrying still, many women are aware of the prevalence of negative perceptions of the menopause amongst the medical and nursing profession. For feminists particularly, the menopause is a political struggle seeking to redefine society's views on older women and their position and opportunities in later life. They feel, often quite rightly, that self-help, gathering the right information and offering mutual support is a better solution compared to the use of inappropriate drug therapy when hormones are used indiscriminately.

Enlightened Attitudes

An alternative way of looking at the menopause is to see it as the next natural stage in any woman's physical development. According to ancient Greek philosophy, each woman's life undergoes several natural phases including puberty, menstruation, pregnancy, childbirth and the menopause. The latter is a calm stage of her life, a time when she is free of the responsibilities of child bearing and child rearing, a period when she finally has time to concentrate on herself and on the creativity and independence which this freedom brings. In many other cultures, the negative menopausal stereotype does not exist. In Japan, for example, there is apparently no word in their language for a hot flush as it appears that very few women experience these adverse symptoms. This is almost certainly because of the high intake of phytoestrogens from natural ingredients in their staple diet, but Japanese women do not share our concept of the menopause either. For them the end of menstruation is of little cultural significance. Instead of the menopause, they describe something known as *Konenki*, a natural stage in life associated with ageing but which is linked to changing function within the autonomic nervous system rather than to oestrogen deficiency. The autonomic nervous system is that part of our nervous system which operates beyond our voluntary control but which is responsible for our response to stress; it controls our capacity to relax and respond to the changing environment around us. In other cultures too, the menopause is seen much more as a natural event taking place as part of the normal ageing process which is not life-threatening, which is not abnormal and which is not in need of pharmaceutical correction or other intervention.

Professionals working in scientific fields other than traditional medicine, for example anthropologists, clinical psychologists, sociologists and epidemiologists, are much more likely to adopt a more positive and philosophical approach to the menopause. Anthropologists, for example, point out that the menopause could in fact confer an evolutionary advantage to women in that by preventing further childbirth it frees women to devote more time to existing children and to create a tighter, healthier and more unified family around them. Sociologists are puzzled to find a medical willingness to replace hormones to treat menopausal symptoms, but a reluctance to offer fertility treatment at the same time. When certain doctors have done this (notably one particular professor who offers egg donation IVF to women up to the age of 65 or thereabouts), they are ridiculed by their colleagues. Psychologists claim that this panders to the common notion within society at large that keeping women young and feminine through hormone treatment is all very well, but encouraging them to continue to be sexually active and have babies is not. Epidemiologists are aware that one of the reasons for the menopause having such a bad press is that only the views of women undergoing severe problems are ever represented. When surveys are conducted within the community as a whole, rather than in hospital clinics where only the very worst sufferers of symptoms are gathered, attitudes towards the menopause are much more positive. In fact, overall, most women have a fairly uneventful menopause with the majority experiencing a few short-lived adverse effects, and some blissfully sailing through menopausal waters with not a care in the world.

Misdiagnosis of the Menopause

I have also found in my own experience in general practice that many women suffering from so-called menopausal symptoms are in fact encountering problems due to other unrelated medical conditions or environmental factors. Depression, so often thought to be the result of 'the change of life', frequently has other root causes such as strains within the family, worries about children who are growing up, and altered expectations for the future. There may be concerns about employment and work, about a relationship with an employer or doubts about whether someone wishes to continue to work at all. Anaemia, thyroid disorders and other physical complaints can often manifest themselves at this time of life, and may be diagnosed incorrectly by physicians and nurses alike as a manifestation of the menopause. The physical symptoms commonly associated with the menopause can have alternative explanations. Research studies have shown that hot flushes, one of the commonest of all menopausal symptoms, can often be relieved through the use of placebos in clinical trials, suggesting that relaxation itself and the fact that care and support is being provided can be as effective as medication. All these factors suggest that in some cases better understanding, support and employment prospects may be just as effective if not more so than the provision of HRT.

Positive Attitude

Positive mental attitude is important in every situation and it is especially important in the menopause. Each and every woman will have a different experience of the menopause and those who have severe symptoms will require help, while others who are untroubled may be quite happy to cope with things on their own. But even those women who do require help should not feel threatened by any kind of appropriate therapeutic intervention and need not abandon their constructive and positive thoughts as they look to their change of life.

The concept of a multi-dimensional personality is central to this. We all have facets of different personalities within us. We are not just a serious person at work, a playful parent at home, the romantic person with our lover or the caring person with those who need our support. We are people who incorporate all these characteristics and we can reflect any of these facets of our nature at any given time. The emotional aspect brought about by any change in a woman's hormones is often overlooked in contemporary Western society. Alterations in mood and personality are natural but there are pressures in society which aim to bring about sameness, to produce personalities which are always rational, always reliable, reasonable and level. There is an innate resistance to change. However, positive change and individual growth is natural and good as well as being feminine – this is what having a change for the better is all about.

One of the things which can make the menopause more acceptable is adequate preparation for it. Just as people may be prepared for retirement or for redundancy, women can be presented with facts about the menopause in a supportive way. If retirement and redundancy are presented as the beginning of the end, people are liable to feel depressed. However, if they have worked their whole lives with a view to having enough money to fulfil their dreams and ambitions when they finally retire, they can look forward to retirement with enthusiasm. Similarly if they have been in a dead-end job working purely for the money, redundancy can be a god send, offering the chance to move on and explore other avenues. The menopause is no different. If only women can learn that hot flushes and emotional ups and downs are likely to be worse before their periods stop rather than after, they might not look upon them with such confusion. If only insomnia and feelings of anxiety whilst lying awake in bed at night could be regarded not as a medical condition but as a natural sign that the menopause is near, it would be easier to come to terms with. The problem is that, just like with bereavement, nobody in our society wants to talk about the menopause, it is an event we would rather shut away from our consciousness and never mention. It is something associated with awkwardness, and difficulty. But rather than seeing it in this light, we should promote it as a journey towards individual freedom, a chance to be more creative and independent. It is a time when women can look forward to a love life without fear of pregnancy, and freedom from the burden of responsibility for children and child rearing. It is a time when, after many years, none of the inconveniences associated with menstruation need be suffered and when the woman need no longer be bound by her role as mother, housekeeper, wife or lover. Anthropologist Margaret Mead even referred to the vigour and energy attendant on the time after the menopause as 'post-menopausal zest'.

Mention the word 'change' to anybody and they very often associate it with stress. Change can certainly be stressful particularly if it is unexpected, unwanted and misunderstood. But stress for one person can simply mean an exciting challenge to somebody else. Provided the menopause is looked upon as a fresh challenge, a new start and as a time to be welcomed in many ways, it can be a stage in a woman's life to be anticipated gladly.

Oestrogen is Not the Be All and End All

Culturally many women have regarded oestrogen as the 'feminine hormone'; they believe that without it after the menopause they will lose all sexuality and femininity. Physiologically it is thought that some women feel less independent just prior to ovulation at the mid-point of their menstrual cycle, when oestrogen levels are at their highest. Anthropologists believe this makes women more sensitive to the needs of others and more aware of their sexuality and the need to find a supportive partner and mate. Some believe that certain women who have particularly high levels of circulating oestrogen are generally more likely to be dependent on others for approval and support. For them it is their co-dependent relationships with others that make them characteristically feminine. Often such individuals initially dread the thought of the menopause as it could threaten their femininity, disrupt their dependence on others and deprive them of one of the founding rocks of their very existence. Ironically, however, many are surprised and thrilled that with their new-found independence and freedom they feel totally complete in themselves for the first time in their entire lives. At this stage many women become aware of and intensify their intuition and spirituality. Now they can follow their own desires regarding education, career and pastimes. This entry into senior womanhood can bring with it a new wisdom and comfort. Women can feel exhilarated by no longer being trapped by many of the social and cultural expectations thrust upon them, and by becoming older but wiser women with the courage to speak their truth. With declining oestrogen levels, a proportionately higher level of testosterone in turn stimulates the emotional and spiritual development of the more masculine side of post-menopausal women, so that those parts of their personalities endow them with the courage to become more independent, self-assertive and powerful. This post-menopausal time can be positive, offering a potential for growth and opportunities for change on all fronts – in careers, hobbies and, sometimes, partners. Many women's groups are available for help and support, and counselling can be of benefit too. It is always worth remembering that in many cultures, older women are regarded as sages and matriarchs, preserving the traditional wisdom of the tribe. Hold your head high as you make this spiritual transition.

CHAPTER TWO

THE MENOPAUSE AND THE PERIMENOPAUSE

What do they mean?

One of the reasons for so much confusion about the menopause is that different people take it to mean different things. There is not even any universal consensus on what it should be called. Many still refer to it simply as 'the change', some call it 'the menopause' or 'the climacteric', and recently the word perimenopause has been increasingly bandied about. What do they signify and do they all describe the same condition?

The word *menopause* literally means the cessation of all menstrual periods. It occurs on the very last day of the very last period, and in practice its exact date can only be accurately confirmed in hindsight. At the time you cannot know for sure that you will not experience further menstruation in the future. You cannot predict this will be your last definite cycle. However, you will for some time almost certainly have noticed certain symptoms leading up to your last menstrual period. These might include irregular, frequent or prolonged periods and cycles, hot flushes, night sweats and insomnia. These are caused by a train of hormonal changes and events gradually occurring over a time span of several months or even years, and which precede and inevitably culminate in your final menstrual period. During this time you can be regarded as perimenopausal, or in other words experiencing the characteristic symptoms which take place 'around the time of' the menopause itself.

The *climacteric* is a less commonly used word which in many medical dictionaries is defined as 'the turn of life – an age at which a person's physical powers begin to decline'. This, however, is an unnecessarily negative description and one from which the more colloquial and certainly more neutral description 'change of life' has evolved.

Confused? I'm Not Surprised

You could be forgiven for thinking that with so much written and talked about the menopause, any woman would instinctively know whether she is experiencing the condition or not. But actually it is not always that easy. Many of the signs and symptoms of the menopause can be incredibly similar to those of other conditions so, for example, its psychological manifestations may be confused with anxiety or depression, and its physical symptoms such as weight change with a thyroid disorder. Occasionally, more than one disorder can occur at the same time adding still further to diagnostic uncertainty and confusion. The consequences attendant on either you yourself, or worse still your doctor, confusing the two can be serious. Incorrect advice or treatment may be handed out with the resultant deterioration of symptoms. In other instances a comparatively young woman can have a particularly premature menopause, a possibility she may never have entertained for a moment, quite reasonably attributing her missed periods to stress or dietary change. She might well remain blissfully unaware of the real situation for some considerable time. In most cases, however, you will know or at least have a strong suspicion that you are menopausal. If you are around the age of 50, your periods have become unpredictable and you have noticed distinct hot flushes for some time, this will undoubtedly be the case.

But what does the word menopause really mean and why does it happen? The change of life is a term everyone understands. This change in each woman's life will be individual and unique but a change in one way or another it will certainly be. Provided that change is a positive one, *a change for the better* that is, at the end of the day it does not really matter what it is called.

Basically you become perimenopausal when the supply of eggs in your ovaries begins to run out and when the levels of the female sex hormone oestrogen start to fall. The diminishing number of remaining eggs then mature only irregularly so that as the menopause proper approaches the length of the menstrual cycles begins to become erratic and the periods themselves become unpredictable and irregular. Although this can happen earlier, it usually starts over the age of 40 and then becomes increasingly noticeable as time goes by. The menopause itself takes place when the ovaries have totally exhausted their supply of functional eggs. This occurs at an average age of 51, but again it can happen earlier – sometimes much earlier, if a menopause is premature. The symptoms women experience during the perimenopause or menopause will vary greatly between individuals, as revealed in later chapters. To understand more completely when and why these changes happen, the basic reproductive anatomy and the normal menstrual cycle need to be described in greater detail, and the various hormones which play a part need to be more fully explained.

Understanding the Basics

Figure 1 shows the important glandular features of female reproduction. A bean-sized area at the base of the brain, the hypothalamus, sits just above the pituitary gland, the hormonal secretions of which interact with each other and in turn influence the function of the ovaries and the lining of the uterus. The uterus itself, the vagina, fallopian tubes and ovaries are seen within the pelvis, with a side-on view of the same pelvic organs and their relationship to one another in Figures 2a and 2b. It will be useful to refer to these diagrams in future chapters. The ovaries in the adult female are about 3.5cm long and resemble soft cream-coloured almonds with an irregular surface. Inside each ovary can be found clusters of specialised cells which surround, protect and nourish the eggs which may one day be released at ovulation time and may, if fertilised by a sperm, develop into an embryo and bring about pregnancy. At birth each baby girl's ovaries already harbour some 450,000 of these follicles. During her lifetime the number of follicles gradually

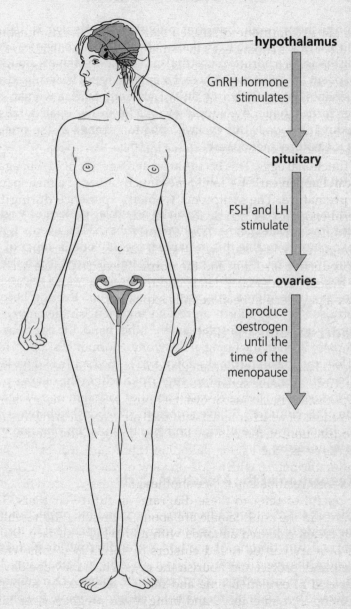

Figure 1 **The glandular factors involved in the normal menstrual cycle**

diminishes overall, but after puberty a single egg is usually released each month from one or other of the two ovaries at the mid-point of a normal menstrual cycle. The egg travels along the adjacent fallopian tube where it may or may not be fertilised and then into the cavity within the womb. Only when a woman is in her forties, when the supply of follicles in her ovaries falls to about 1,000, does this cyclical situation change in the prelude to the natural menopause.

The Normal Menstrual Cycle

Normal menstrual cycles result in a regular pattern of vaginal bleeding which occurs about once a month. The events which take place to enable this to happen include one or other of the two ovaries releasing an egg which travels along the adjacent fallopian tube towards the uterus. Prior to the egg's release the lining of the uterus thickens so that should the egg become fertilised by a sperm it can receive and nourish the embryo. If conception fails to take place on the other hand, the egg does not implant itself in the lining of the womb, hormonal support for it is lost and the lining breaks down and is shed some 14 days later. Thereafter further immature eggs ripen within the ovaries prior to the next one being released another fortnight or so later. So the cycle continues. I have shown the relationship between the proliferation of the uterine lining and ovulation diagrammatically in Figure 3.

Regulation of the Menstrual Cycle

The release of each egg from the ovary and the proliferation of the lining of the womb (endometrium) is dependent in turn on normal functioning of the body's 'endocrine' or glandular system, the overall controller of which is the hypothalamus. This and a tiny pea-sized gland just beneath it, with which it intimately interacts, regulate the menstrual cycle and promote the physiological events which in optimum conditions create the circumstances whereby a possible pregnancy might take place.

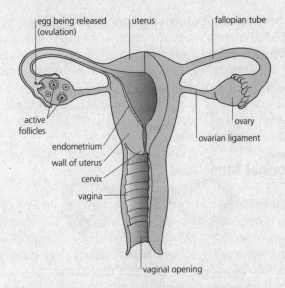

Figure 2a **The female reproductive organs**

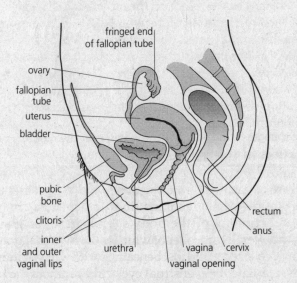

Figure 2b **Side-view of the female reproductive organs within the pelvis**

WATERFORD

Female monthly cycle without fertilisation

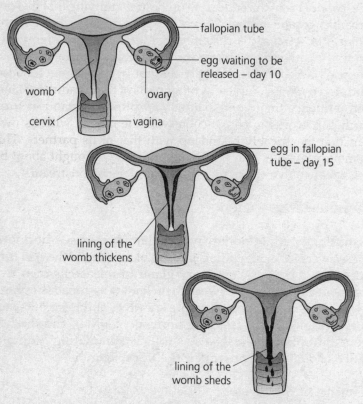

- fallopian tube
- egg waiting to be released – day 10
- womb
- ovary
- cervix
- vagina
- egg in fallopian tube – day 15
- lining of the womb thickens
- lining of the womb sheds

The changes in the lining of the womb over the monthly cycle

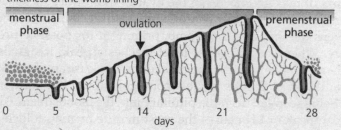

thickness of the womb lining

menstrual phase | ovulation | premenstrual phase

0   5   14   21   28

days

Figure 3

Many medical textbooks still refer to the hypothalamus as being the 'conductor of the endocrine orchestra' implying that this one area has greater influence over the menstrual cycle than any other. But whilst it is certainly true that stress or significant weight change brought about by eating disorders such as anorexia nervosa can seriously disrupt hypothalamic function and stop periods completely, other parts of the glandular system can influence the hypothalamus and pituitary gland in turn. Each part works in conjunction with the others, with its own function inextricably bound up with that of its partners. This communication and interaction is constantly brought about by the release of hormonal messengers into the bloodstream.

Hormone Messengers

A normally functioning hypothalamus releases hormone messengers in regular bursts into the bloodstream; these in turn stimulate the nearby pituitary gland to release its own two hormone messengers, between them known as gonadotrophins. The hypothalamic messengers are known as nothing more fancy than gonadotrophin releasing hormone (GnRH), and the two gonadotrophins themselves as follicle stimulating hormone (FSH) and luteinising hormone (LH). See Figure 1.

Timing of the Cycles

The release of the first hormone, FSH, in turn stimulates the most mature of the egg follicles in the ovaries to produce increasing quantities of another hormone, oestradiol, which directly thickens the lining of the womb, priming it for possible pregnancy. When the oestradiol level reaches a peak, it signals a further response from the hypothalamus to release another burst of GnRH which results in the second gonadotrophin hormone, LH, being secreted from the pituitary into the bloodstream. This sudden peak of LH causes the most mature ovarian follicle to burst, releasing the enclosed egg and completing the process of ovulation.

The ruptured follicle which remains, known as the corpus luteum, then collapses. It becomes yellowish in colour and whilst it still produces a little oestradiol, it now begins to generate the other predominant female sex hormone, progesterone, as well. Progesterone now influences the uterine lining to proliferate even further so that the egg now released can implant more effectively should it become fertilised and conception ensue. At this stage the timing of hormonal events becomes critical. The corpus luteum will only survive a few days and oestrogen and progesterone levels begin to fall as time goes on. Without these two hormones the endometrium cannot survive either and unless pregnancy takes place, major changes soon occur. The lining breaks down and becomes separated from the tissues beneath it. Blood vessels which have developed and proliferated during the first part of the menstrual cycle begin to close down and seal themselves off. Clotted blood and cellular debris collect within the uterine cavity where special enzymes liquify the contents so the contractions of the muscular uterine wall can expel them through the cervix and into the vagina. At this stage, when the period has begun, oestradiol levels are low again and the pituitary gland, sensing this situation through biological negative feedback, responds once more by secreting FSH into the bloodstream thereby commencing another identical cycle. These hormone changes during the menstrual cycle are shown in Figure 4.

Cycles usually continue in this way (with minor aberrations from time to time) between puberty and the menopause, unless pregnancy intervenes. When it does, the lining of the uterus obviously needs to be maintained in order to nourish the embryo and allow permanent implantation, and it clearly could not manage this without hormonal support. In fact it is the embryo itself which prevents menstruation by producing a hormone of its own called human chorionic gonadotrophin which keeps the corpus luteum alive so that it can continue to produce oestrogen and progesterone in sufficient quantities. Within two months of these events, however, the placenta has developed sufficiently to produce enough hormone of its own to take over from the

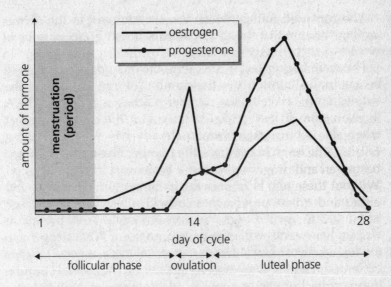

Figure 4 **Hormone changes through the menstrual cycle**

corpus luteum and the pregnancy becomes increasingly viable and less vulnerable to miscarriage as a result. So what happens to this complex hormonal regulation of the menstrual cycle leading up to the menopause and how does it affect periods and fertility?

NATURAL MENOPAUSE

The Prelude to the Natural Menopause

Most women experience their natural menopause between the ages of 48 and 55. Whether or not the old wives' tale is true that a woman can expect to go through her menopause at roughly the same age as her mother did, remains to be scientifically proven, but it does seem to be the case that the average age of the menopause has remained very much the same for several centuries. Unlike the timing of puberty which in recent years has occurred at younger and younger ages, the evolutionary factors determining the onset of the menopause at about 51 seem to have remained surprisingly constant.

The main trigger factor presaging the menopause appears to be gradual diminution in the number of egg follicles in the ovaries until, critically, the number reaches as few as 1,000. A thousand may in fact sound like quite a lot, but considering that when she is born each woman already has a store of about 450,000 follicles in her ovaries, the number remaining is indeed comparatively low. Supposing a woman starts ovulating at puberty when she is 12 and finally stops ovulating near her menopause when she is 52, then she will only ever have released less than 500 ripened eggs. Precious few of the store present at birth in her ovaries will ever have been used. What happens to the rest of them? During each menstrual cycle several follicles become ripe at the same time in response to hormonal stimulation and all but the one which releases an egg then become redundant. Others also gradually disappear over the years, but undoubtedly some other very significant but yet unidentified factors accelerate this process when a woman reaches her forties.

Egg Follicles and Hormones at the Menopause

Not only are fewer and fewer follicles still present in the ovaries as the menopause approaches, but those which do remain become less responsive to hormonal stimulation. Since the pituitary gland recognises this lack of response through the negative feedback mechanism of falling oestrogen levels, it automatically increases its secretion of FSH each month in an attempt to remedy this situation. FSH being secreted into the bloodstream can be measured using laboratory techniques on blood samples, the results showing a distinct rise in level over this perimenopausal period and beyond. At first, the FSH level fluctuates from day to day and cycle to cycle so that in the perimenopausal period a one-off reading can be misleading. Over the course of time, however, and coupled with classic symptoms of the menopause such as hot flushes and night sweats, the blood levels of

FSH increase steadily and significantly. Whilst oestrogen levels fall, LH also rises to a level three to five times what it measured pre-menstrually. These two blood tests (for FSH and LH) are therefore useful indicators to doctors and their women patients in helping to decide whether a woman is in her menopause or at least perimenopausal or not, and what action if any needs to be taken. Whilst FSH levels are raised in this situation the ovarian follicles remain less functional with the result that the normal menstrual cycle may become unpredictable or erratic. Because less oestradiol is secreted by the remaining follicles, the first half of the cycle can become shorter, leading to more frequent periods every 21 days or so. Sometimes eggs are not released at all at mid-cycle time, and the consequence of this is that without a corpus luteum (the follicle sac which remains after ovulation) progesterone is not manufactured; this leads to continued proliferation of the lining of the uterus under the unbalanced influence of oestradiol, and a heavier and possibly delayed period can occur.

Declining Fertility

Logically, if ovulation is taking place less often, fertility is also reduced and whilst contraception is still required (to be on the safe side) in the perimenopause, over a third of women aged 45 and over are almost certainly no longer ovulating. Finally, as the last few ovarian follicles cease to produce oestradiol, the lining of the uterus fails to proliferate in the first part of the menstrual cycle and periods stop altogether. The levels of oestrogen in the blood fall by as much as 80 per cent in the first year following the menopause and the relationship of these levels in the perimenopausal period and beyond can be seen in Figure 5.

Diagnosing the Menopause

By definition a woman is menopausal when she has not had a period for one year. Unfortunately this is unhelpful for women wishing to know where in relation to her perimenopause she

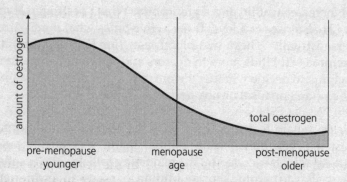

Pre-menopause, oestrogen levels follow a regular pattern
during the menstrual cycle with a surge at mid-cycle
triggering the release of an egg from the ovary (ovulation).
Post-menopause, the ovaries no longer produce maturing eggs,
oestrogen levels fall and the periods cease altogether.

Figure 5 **Oestrogen levels before and after the menopause**

currently is, and it is not helpful whatsoever to a woman who has had a hysterectomy, since her periods have already stopped. It would be delightfully convenient if there was a simple, quick, painless and reliable test that could diagnose with certainty whether a woman is in her menopause or not. Regrettably life is not that easy. We've already seen that symptoms suggesting the menopause, while helpful in their own right, could often be caused by other unrelated medical conditions. Menstrual irregularities may have a number of causes and explanations, and even hot flushes, night sweats or palpitations may well be due to some totally separate medical disorder. If a woman with irregular and heavy periods is encouraged to keep a menstrual diary, however, supplied by her doctor and fully explained to her, it certainly helps to understand the pattern and nature of some of these symptoms. Over a three-month time span the diary charts the days when bleeding occurs, how heavy it is, whether clots are noticed and how much discomfort is experienced. Additional notes can be kept for recording symptoms other than cycle irregularities. Together with blood tests for FSH and LH levels, which for reasons already discussed may not in themselves always be totally reliable, a diagnosis can generally be conclusively reached.

Hormones in the Menopause

If the diagnosis of the menopause is reached by way of blood tests and symptoms, what is it that actually brings about the menopausal symptoms themselves? In the recent past most doctors would have undoubtedly and almost unanimously answered: falling oestrogen levels. Whilst to a very great degree they would have been right and still are, the full answer is not quite as straightforward as all that. Several of the most classic menstrual symptoms, such as hot flushes, night sweats and vaginal dryness, are certainly known to be a direct consequence of oestrogen deficiency. But other symptoms, especially anxiety, insomnia and depression, may well have other explanations and causes and are possibly not related to changing hormone status at all. Long-term complications of the menopause however, notably a greater risk of heart disease and osteoporosis, are inextricably linked to falling oestrogen levels without doubt.

We hear a lot about oestrogen, the predominant female sex hormone, and many myths and prejudices about it have developed as a result of widespread over-simplifications. Contrary to popular belief, oestrogen is by no means the only important hormone in female reproductive physiology and we have already heard about progesterone and its vital role in the normal menstrual cycle. Women also produce testosterone (the 'male' hormone) in small quantities just as men produce oestrogen in small quantities, and each of these naturally occurring steroid hormones have an important function to fulfil in the female body. Certainly oestrogen can be regarded as the feminising hormone and testosterone as one of the masculinising hormones or androgens, but structurally they are all closely related (Figure 6).

The basic steroid molecule consists of four hydrocarbon rings joined together to form the characteristic geometric shape. Only

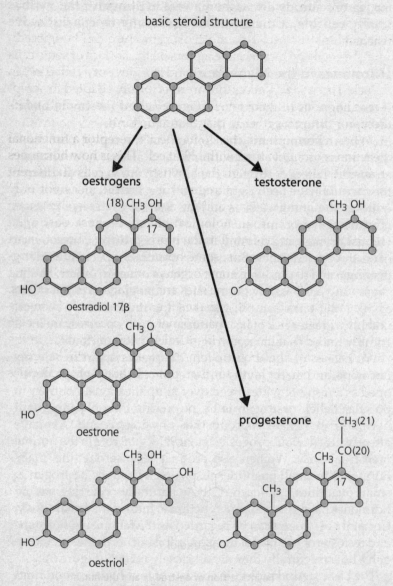

basic steroid structure

oestrogens   testosterone

(18) CH₃ OH   CH₃ OH

HO

oestradiol 17β

CH₃ O

HO

oestrone

CH₃ OH
         OH   progesterone   CH₃(21)
                                                             CO(20)
                                                    CH₃ 17
         CH₃

HO   O

oestriol

Figure 6 **The chemical structure of sex hormones**

minor alterations, in terms of attached side chains consisting of oxygen, hydrogen or carbon atoms, distinguish the various hormones from one another and confer upon them a distinctive molecular structure. This molecular structure can be immediately recognised by special receptors on the surface of some cells into which it can snugly fit like a hand in a glove or a coded key in a lock. These special receptors are specifically adapted to accept some hormones but not others. Figure 7 shows oestradiol and its receptor fitting together in diagrammatic form.

When a hormone attaches to its specific receptor a functional reaction is brought about within that cell. This is how hormones transmit messages through the bloodstream to cells at different sites within the body. Oestrogen, for example, does not only thicken the lining of the womb by attaching to receptors there, but brings about other biological effects because oestrogen receptors can also be found in the brain, pituitary, breast, heart and skeleton. Furthermore, some hormones are capable of triggering some receptors in some organs but not in others, leading to stimulation of cells at some sites and total inactivity at others. The hand in glove analogy makes it easy to see how hormone therapy works since a man-made or naturally occurring molecule which is identical or nearly identical to hormones made in the body can also bring about cellular change as it too can be recognised as the correct hand for that glove. In addition, molecules

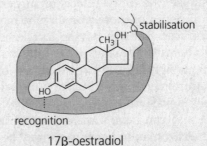

17β-oestradiol

Figure 7 **The interaction of oestradiol and the human oestrogen receptor**

which closely resemble the correct hand for the glove or the correct key for the lock may be only partially recognised by a receptor, causing blocking of that receptor site without bringing about any cellular change at all, but with inhibition of the usual action of the hormone made by the body. Both naturally occuring plant oestrogens (phytoestrogens) and synthetic hormones made by drug companies may work on a receptor site in this way and bring about either deliberate or unwanted effects. One example of this is the synthetic hormone ethinyl-oestradiol used in the contraceptive pill, the effect of which is much more potent than that of natural oestradiol and which can therefore influence the menstrual cycle to the extent that it can prevent ovulation completely and prevent unplanned pregnancy.

PREMATURE MENOPAUSE

Most women, as we have already said, experience the menopause between the ages of 48 and 55. However, a significant number of women have their menopause earlier, and recent research has given us a much better idea of the numbers involved. It seems that one in a hundred women develop spontaneous ovarian failure before the age of 40 and one in a thousand suffer the same fate before they even reach 30. These figures do not take into account either those women having an earlier menopause due to the effects of surgery to remove the ovaries and/or uterus, or those women who have had a medical menopause induced through having to take chemotherapy or undergo radiotherapy for malignant conditions. Overall, we are not talking about significantly large numbers of women undergoing a premature menopause, but for those who do, it can be a psychologically devastating event, especially if it occurs before the age of 30, and can have a major impact on that woman's quality of life. A woman in her thirties may be acutely focused on the idea of starting a family or having another child if she already has a family, and being told future fertility is out of the question or at best highly unlikely can be a considerable blow.

Symptoms of Premature Menopause

Unlike those women who have a normally timed natural menopause, only about 50 per cent of women experiencing a
premature menopause are aware of symptoms of hot flushes and
night sweats. Even those who do may well not attribute them to
the menopause as this would be totally unexpected at their relatively young age. So the first indication that anything is wrong
may be irregular and unpredictable periods. It is this development which eventually means that a woman goes to see the doctor
for further investigation and help. Between them, the patient and
her doctor will initially look at more common causes of absent
or infrequent periods, the top of the list question being could she
be pregnant? If this is not the case and pregnancy is ruled out
with a straightforward pregnancy test, the most likely reason for
absent periods would probably be any major recent weight
change. People on crash diets or those who have become
anorexic, for example, and even women who are considerably
overweight and obese can often experience menstrual irregularities for this reason. Sometimes moving away to university,
moving house or experiencing increased stress at work or in
relationships can cause enough emotional upset to temporarily
disturb the normal function of the hypothalamus and pituitary
gland too. In addition, vigorous exercise or intense athletic
training can have similar effects as can taking the oral contraceptive pill, which in a few women can delay the onset of periods
once the pill is discontinued. Less commonly, a benign swelling
in the pituitary gland can develop and disturb pituitary and
ovarian function. So the possibility of premature ovarian failure
is often one of the last possibilities to be considered.

Medical tests would probably include amongst other things
hormone level measurements, magnetic resonance imaging
(MRI) scans and ultrasound tests. Hormone measurements are
usually carried out first as they are quickly arranged, convenient
and relatively inexpensive. FSH levels are elevated in premature
ovarian failure because the lack of ovarian follicles and the
decreased amount of circulating oestradiol in the bloodstream

stimulates the pituitary to produce more FSH in an effort to make the ovaries respond. There is less to be gained from measuring oestradiol levels in the bloodstream as these generally only fall to a low level much later on. Even then, a single FSH level might not be diagnostic. There is usually a slight increase in the production of FSH prior to each normal monthly ovulation anyway and just in case the measurement proves to be elevated because it has been taken at this pre-ovulation time, a repeat test is important to assess the true picture. In other words, the FSH test for premature menopause is not as definitive as a pregnancy test or a test for anaemia since the result may be variable and open to interpretation. It can, however, contribute to the overall assessment and sometimes a significantly elevated FSH level in a young woman who is not having any periods, particularly if it is above 40 international units per litre (40 iu/l) persistently, may be diagnostic.

When a woman gives blood for FSH measurements, she will probably also have three other hormone measurements carried out, for thyroid function, LH and prolactin levels. Abnormal thyroid function can certainly influence periods and can also induce weight changes and alterations in appetite, and lead to heat intolerance or feeling the cold. Normal thyroid function test results more or less rule out the possibility of a thyroid disorder. Since it is known that LH levels increase after the menopause, a significantly elevated level in conjunction with a raised FSH level is highly suggestive of a premature menopause in a younger woman.

Doctors also measure prolactin, another hormone produced by the pituitary gland. Prolactin is secreted by this gland in greater quantities during breast-feeding and since prolactin can inhibit and alter the normal menstrual cycle, resulting in temporary infertility, knowledge of the prolactin level is important in the investigation of premature menopause. Prolactin levels can also be increased as a result of taking certain medications, of being subjected to intense stress and occasionally as a result of developing a pituitary adenoma, a benign cystic growth within the gland itself.

Supposing hormone measurements suggest a premature menopause, what happens next? The general practitioner will by this stage almost certainly have referred a woman patient to the gynaecologist. The gynaecologist in turn will wish to know whether there is genuinely a lack of follicles in the ovaries or whether there are follicles present but they have simply become unresponsive to the gonadotrophin hormones secreted by the pituitary gland. In the past the first test would have been an ovarian biopsy requiring a general anaesthetic and a surgical procedure to remove a small sample of ovarian tissue for visual analysis under the microscope. These days it is much more likely that a woman will have an ultrasound scan in the first instance because it is non-invasive and quick. The woman attends when the bladder is full so that the ovaries become more accessible for the test. A little oil is poured on to the skin over the abdomen and sound-waves are transmitted through it by way of a small transducer. The echoes of these sound-waves are picked up on a mini computer enabling a picture to be built up of the ovaries and of the number of follicles therein. The scan shows up follicles as tiny dark spots on a background of opaque ovarian tissue. Sometimes it is obvious that there are simply very few follicles there, but at other times we see plenty of follicles but ones which are clearly not responding to hormonal stimulation, a condition known as resistant ovary syndrome.

Why Does Premature Menopause Occur?

There may be many reasons for a lack of ovarian follicles. We know that baby girls when they are born already have something like 450,000 follicles present in their ovaries. There are normally plenty to tide her over her reproductive years and to last until she reaches the age at which she can expect a normal natural menopause. However, if ovarian development is detrimentally influenced by environmental factors at any time, follicles may be destroyed. Ovarian surgery, hysterectomy, cancer treatment, viral infections such as mumps, or even autoimmune disease (where the body's own antibodies for some reason become programmed to destroy its own ovarian tissue) may all damage the ovarian follicles. There are also a number of genetic and chromosomal abnormalities which may play a part in bringing about premature menopause. In many cases the underlying cause may never become clear although it seems that whatever factors bring about the accelerated loss of follicles in women having a normally timed natural menopause, they kick in at a much earlier age in women who experience a premature menopause.

Treatment

Perhaps the most important aspect of treatment is to consider the emotional impact of the diagnosis and its implications and to offer help and support at this time. Not only is the woman's fertility seriously threatened, but she is likely to suffer all the short-term and long-term complications of the menopause at a much younger age than other women. She may well need treatment to ease these symptoms and to protect her long term against brittle bone disease (osteoporosis) and heart disease. In this situation combined hormone replacement therapy offers considerable benefits and is often recommended. The combined form of hormone replacement therapy using both oestrogen *and* progestogen is important as the lining of the womb needs to be protected against the unopposed action of oestrogen alone. This is explained more fully in later chapters.

If the patient wishes to have children in the future the options for treatment can be discussed. Possibilities for fertility treatment include the use of clomiphene which can be given to stimulate ovulation (even in premature ovarian failure) and this therapy is usually worth trying first, prior to other options such as egg donation in-vitro fertilisation. Here, eggs from another woman (donor) may be fertilised in the test-tube by the woman's own partner's sperm to produce a number of embryos. Then, either two or three embryos can be transferred back into the woman's womb in the hope of achieving a pregnancy. At the same time many other embryos may be frozen and stored in the event that the first course of egg donation IVF treatment may not be successful. There are many difficulties and pitfalls associated with this kind of fertility treatment however, and women undergoing a premature menopause need to be fully counselled, not least about the emotional hardships, financial implications and time involved. There is also a significantly high failure rate. However, the very hope that it remains feasible to undergo such treatment and start a family at some time in the future can be enormously reassuring to the woman concerned. In an ideal world, a good, caring GP and specialist gynaecologist will spend time with a woman and her partner in this situation. They will know that she may well be going through a form of bereavement reaction to her infertility and that she may feel distressed because she perceives herself to be 'old before her time'. It may also be that without proper understanding, her partner, who himself may desperately wish to start a family, finds the woman's situation difficult to accept. Pressure from other members of her family, and the nagging feeling that she may have let potential grandparents down in not being able to have children are all notions which warrant discussion and counselling.

SURGICAL MENOPAUSE

Quite commonly, women do not have a natural menopause but have one which is brought about as a result of medical or surgical treatment for other conditions. In each case there are short-term and long-term implications for the woman, encompassing not only the anticipated symptoms and signs of the menopause but relating to fertility as well. The provision of adequate information, consultation and choice is therefore imperative.

Ovarian Problems

Figure 8 shows the normal anatomy of the ovary with the presence of maturing ovarian follicles and a corpus luteum. Recurrent ovarian cysts, endometriosis or ovarian cancer would all warrant surgical removal of diseased ovaries. Cysts are the

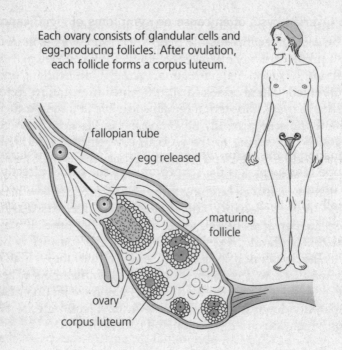

Each ovary consists of glandular cells and
egg-producing follicles. After ovulation,
each follicle forms a corpus luteum.

fallopian tube

egg released

maturing
follicle

ovary

corpus luteum

Figure 8 **The anatomy of the ovary**

commonest reason for having ovarian surgery and when a
woman's symptoms are suggestive of ovarian dysfunction,
ultrasound scans often reveal the obvious enlargement of these
organs. Identifiable cysts may be solid or filled with fluid, there
may be several of them as opposed to just one or two, and of course
they may be present in both ovaries as opposed to just the one.

But not all ovarian cysts need to be removed. In the majority
of cases (about 95 per cent) they are benign and not cancerous.
Many ovarian cysts also disappear without requiring treatment.
The commonest type is the follicular cyst where the egg-
producing follicle of the ovary enlarges and fills with fluid. Cysts
can also arise from the corpus luteum, the yellow mass of tissue
which develops after ovulation has taken place. Other kinds of
ovarian cysts include solid dermoid cysts (containing skin
tissue) and malignant cysts which may be either solid or fluid

filled. Ovarian cysts often cause no symptoms of significance until the later stages when abdominal discomfort, pain during love-making or menstrual irregularities may occur. These include absent periods, heavy or painful periods. Also, occasional abdominal pain, nausea and fever can arise if an ovarian cyst twists on its stalk and cuts off its blood supply or if a cyst ruptures. Cysts may be found during a routine internal examination, during ultrasound scanning or at laparoscopy, an examination of the abdominal cavity using a special fibre-optic telescope which enables the surgeon to see the ovary directly. Quite often it is only the cyst itself which needs to be removed, especially if it is small, but much larger ones and solid cysts, particularly malignant ones, will generally necessitate removal of the entire ovary, an operation known as oophorectomy.

Other reasons for surgically removing either an entire ovary or both ovaries include conditions such as endometriosis, whereby the cells which normally line the uterus escape along the fallopian tubes and establish themselves on the surface of the ovary and even on the outside of the fallopian tubes and the uterus, bladder and other abdominal organs. At the end of the menstrual cycle, at period time, this tissue then bleeds along with the rest of the endometrial cells still lying within the womb, which leads to abdominal discomfort, pain during intercourse and subfertility.

Hysterectomy

Sometimes entirely healthy ovaries are surgically removed, particularly during a hysterectomy carried out because of heavy periods or the presence of fibroids, although in this situation the procedure is somewhat controversial. In the region of 90,000 hysterectomies are carried out every year in the UK and in some 14 per cent removal of both ovaries takes place even though they are healthy and free of disease. The surgeon takes the view in these instances that while the womb is being removed, there is also an opportunity to remove the ovaries since fertility is no longer required and since their hormonal function can be taken over by hormone replacement therapy. The benefits are that any potential cancer arising in the ovaries at a later date, which could seriously threaten the life of that patient, can be avoided. This is particularly true, they would argue, since there is no adequate screening test for ovarian cancer, even in women with a strong family history of it, and because symptoms of ovarian cancer are only noticed by women themselves in the very late stages of the disease when curative treatment may no longer be possible.

Bearing in mind that more women die in Britain from ovarian cancer than from cervical cancer, for which we have a screening campaign that attracts so much publicity, such opinions carry weight. However, other gynaecologists and many women themselves take the view that without a positive family history of ovarian cancer, the risk of ovarian cancer developing is low, especially after the age of 55, and that statistically large numbers of women would have to undergo the unnecessary loss of both their ovaries in order to prevent a single case of ovarian cancer in low risk women.

Clearly in this situation there are pros and cons, which makes it extremely important that women are fully informed before they consent to such drastic surgical intervention. Suffice it to say that in the UK, 85 per cent of gynaecologists have stated that they would generally remove a woman's ovaries if she was already post-menopausal. As in all cases of treatment, the benefits must be weighed against the potential risks. Younger women who have their ovaries removed, unless they take hormone replacement therapy afterwards, have a two-fold increased risk of developing coronary heart disease as a result of the operation, and their life expectancy can be expected to be reduced by up to five years. Hormone replacement therapy offsets this detrimental effect, but many women remain to be convinced that HRT is as acceptable as the natural hormones secreted by the ovaries. But difficult decisions like these often have to be faced. In the UK, of women who undergo a hysterectomy one in 20 are under the age of 40, and one in 50 are under the age of 35. In some of these cases the ovaries themselves will harbour problems and require removal anyway, so decisions are made easier, but for younger women having a hysterectomy with healthy ovaries, oophorectomy is certainly not usually performed, and even for women aged 45–49 in this situation, less than a quarter of British gynaecologists recommend it. In fact, some medical studies have suggested that hysterectomy itself can promote an earlier menopause than would otherwise have occurred, with some women experiencing it up to four years earlier than usual.

Informed Consent

In view of all the implications, any woman contemplating surgery must be made aware of all the relevant facts and figures and understand completely all the pros and cons before agreeing to subject herself to an operation. Without such 'informed consent' no surgeon is legally permitted to remove a woman's ovaries or any other organs for that matter during hysterectomy.

Symptoms of Surgical Menopause

The clinical effect of having both ovaries removed is a surgical menopause with a fairly dramatic onset of symptoms in most cases. Hot flushes and night sweats are likely to occur within a matter of days, with insomnia, generalised aches and pains and headaches quite likely in addition. But symptoms are by no means a certainty, and some follow-up studies have suggested that about a third of patients experience no symptoms whatsoever. In those that do, however, it is believed to be the very sudden and significant fall in oestradiol levels which causes the problems. In the wake of these declining levels, the pituitary gland produces a surge of FSH which is easily detectable through biochemical measurement in blood tests. The hypothalamus is also alerted by such a rapid diminution in ovarian hormone levels and activity here is believed to influence the thermo-regulatory centre in an adjacent part of the brain. The resultant stimulation of the autonomic nervous system which governs temperature control throughout the body is thought to be a major factor in the initiation of menopausal symptoms, particularly hot flushes and night sweats. Interestingly it may well be that larger women tend to have an easier time of it after surgical menopause than their thinner counterparts as their body fat is capable of producing certain types of oestrogen, namely oestrone, in its own right.

Surgical removal of the ovaries also leads to a significant decline in levels of testosterone and its androgenic derivatives with a sudden drop of up to 50 per cent occurring as a consequence. During a natural menopause on the other hand, the decline is only about 20 per cent because post-menopausally the ovaries are still able to produce some testosterone. As a result, a surgically induced menopause can sometimes lead to a reduction in libido and sex drive. Coupled with notable vaginal dryness caused by oestrogen deficiency, this can lead to discomfort or even pain during intercourse, and adds to the distress linked to the surgery.

To avoid these symptoms and the long-term consequences of a premature menopause such as osteoporosis and heart disease, the immediate use of HRT is therefore recommended. Without a uterus, oestrogen-only HRT is suitable and there are many types to choose from, including a regime which incorporates small doses of testosterone if loss of libido is a problem. Some women find it difficult to decide initially which of the various options they wish to take, and may for this reason elect to have an HRT implant inserted at the time of surgery which will bide them over for several months until they have thought more carefully about what treatment they might prefer in the future. Women who have suffered medical conditions relating to their ovaries are also eligible for HRT in most instances. There is a small risk of recurrence of endometriosis if hormones are taken as these will obviously stimulate any endometrial cells remaining, just as they would the lining of the womb if it were still present. But the chances of this happening have been estimated at a mere 5 per cent and if opposed oestrogen is prescribed (where progestogens are given as well), or if an alternative such as tibolone is recommended, no problems with recurrences should be experienced. Some of the newer 'selective oestrogen receptor modulators' (SERMS) can also be considered in this situation as they have no effect on endometrial tissue and also help protect against osteoporosis. They do not offer much in the way of relief for the immediate menopausal symptoms, however, so their use at present has limitations.

The overall rationale for recommending HRT after a surgical menopause is therefore very strong. So much so that providing there are no medical reasons for not doing so, the vast majority of gynaecologists steadfastly advise women to take HRT in this situation, a quarter advising its use indefinitely. However there is a worrying gulf between medical expediency and what actually happens at the present time. The National Osteoporosis Society (NOS) found that of the 25 per cent of their members who had had a surgically induced menopause, some 75 per cent had never been offered HRT. Also, apart from women who had undergone oophorectomy because of ovarian cancer, very few women who were started on HRT in hospital were ever properly followed up and reappraised to find out how they were getting on with their HRT. This practice, or rather lack of it, leaves much to be desired and is medically unsatisfactory, as adjustments to treatment are often required. Consequently a formal statement has been published recently by the Royal College of Obstetricians and Gynaecologists, the Royal College of General Practitioners, and the National Osteoporosis Society in conjunction with one another to strongly recommend regular monitoring of all women prescribed HRT after a surgical menopause either in hospital clinics or in the GP setting. It is immaterial who carries out the monitoring and where it is done, the important thing is that it *is* carried out and on a regular basis.

The Prospect of Infertility

In terms of fertility most women having oophorectomy will have a hysterectomy at the same time, the only options then remaining open in terms of enjoying children are adoption or fostering. If the uterus *is* left intact, however, the possibility remains of having eggs removed prior to ovarian surgery so that they may be fertilised by the partner's sperm and stored in frozen embryo form. Another possibility is egg donation IVF where another woman's eggs are used in a similar way.

MEDICAL MENOPAUSE

A medical menopause occurs as a result of side effects of medical treatment for life-threatening conditions. In younger women malignancies such as leukaemia (cancer of the bone marrow), lymphoma (cancer of the lymph glands) or breast cancer are treated with combinations of radiotherapy and chemotherapy in an attempt to destroy the rapidly dividing cells which are cancerous. These are the best treatments currently available and they achieve a cure in many cases, especially if treatment is begun early enough. Regrettably, however, these treatments have a non-specific action and damage all cells they come into contact with, not just the cancerous ones. It is the price that has to be paid. It is the rapidly dividing cells which are the most vulnerable to their action and unfortunately the actively dividing cells of the ovarian follicles fall into that category also. The longer treatment lasts and the bigger the dose of drugs or radiation used, the more likely it is that all follicles within the ovaries will be destroyed. Younger women have most resistance to this side effect of cancer treatment as one might expect as their ovaries start off with greater numbers of follicles, and pregnancy is not at all unheard of among women who have undergone such therapy at a later stage.

If you are concerned about your future fertility before you embark on such treatment, your dosage of radiotherapy can be deliberately reduced and your ovaries protected from the direction of the radiotherapy beam, especially if the organ targeted for treatment is located at a more distant site in your body. Other options include the removal of eggs from your ovaries prior to treatment so that fertilisation with your partner's sperm can be organised in vitro with storage of frozen embryos for further use. The very latest option involves the complete surgical removal of your ovaries before any treatment with a view to having them transplanted back into your own body at some stage in the future when all detrimental side effects of potentially damaging cancer treatment are deemed to have disappeared. This procedure currently remains experimental and at the time of writing no woman who has undergone it has resumed periods or become pregnant. High expectations of this technique will certainly prevail for the future.

In terms of treatment for symptoms occurring as a result of medical menopause, in most instances 'combined' HRT will be advisable. This is because oestrogen needs to be opposed and balanced by progestogen so that the lining of the intact womb does not overproliferate and lead to the potentially pre-malignant condition known as endometrial hyperplasia. There are no concerns relating to the reactivation of malignant conditions such as leukaemia or Hodgkins Disease by HRT because these cancers, unlike breast or uterine cancers, are not hormone related.

CHAPTER 3

PHYSICAL SYMPTOMS AND
HOW TO TREAT THEM

There are a large number of symptoms commonly associated with the menopause and this chapter deals with the physical ones. Before I launch into a relatively long list, it is important to realise that not all women will experience all of these symptoms, and a lucky few will never experience any of them. Overall, however, the majority of women will be able to identify to some extent with some of the symptoms which are looked at in this chapter. Knowing that you are not alone, and understanding what causes your symptoms and how they can best be treated, may be very helpful. The symptoms include the following:

hot flushes, night sweats and palpitations
irregular periods
vaginal dryness
putting on weight
urinary problems
dry skin and wrinkles
thinning hair
headaches and migraines
decreased muscle tone
joint and muscle pains and fatigue
constipation and irritable bowel syndrome

HOT FLUSHES AND NIGHT SWEATS

Hot flushes are amongst the commonest menopausal symptoms of all with something like 80 per cent of all women in Britain and in other Westernised countries suffering from them. Although not all menopausal symptoms are related to falling oestrogen levels at this time, hot flushes and night sweats undoubtedly are. They are often described as a sensation of warmth or even intense heat during which time your skin will flush and perspiration will occur. Sometimes the perspiration may be visible and the sensation of heat can lead to rapid cooling of the skin resulting in a chill or frisson. The pulse rate rises, the skin temperature increases and these changes can occur up to 30 times a day in severe cases. The flush usually begins on the chest or face radiating out thereafter all over the body. This may last a brief 30 seconds or be quite protracted and last several minutes in some cases. Palpitations, a feeling of pounding of the heart, of missed heartbeats or a fluttery sensation within the chest may also occur and last up to an hour or so.

Hot flushes and night sweats tend to begin at around the age of 47 or 48, usually persisting for two to three years. In some women hot flushes may occur much earlier, in the late thirties or early forties and can continue for five to fifteen years. When you start having hot flushes they often begin during the week before your period is due when oestrogen levels begin to fall naturally. Later, as the menopause nears, hot flushes can occur at any stage during the menstrual cycle. The majority of women will no longer have hot flushes of any significance beyond three years post-menopausally but up to 25 per cent will still have occasional flushes for more than five years beyond the menopause and an unlucky few will still experience them for the rest of their lives. Women are likely to seek their doctor's advice when these symptoms become much more intense and disruptive. More than 15 per cent of post-menopausal women say that their hot flushes are frequent and severe, rendering their lives uncomfortable and making them irritable and tetchy.

The underlying cause of hot flushes is 'oestrogen withdrawal', in other words a drop in circulating oestrogen level in the bloodstream. Even women who are young and have just had a baby can suffer hot flushes when the previously high levels of oestrogen suddenly begin falling post-natally. At the menopause, since the hypothalamus at the base of the brain is stimulated to become more active when oestrogen levels fall, its increased activity in turn stimulates the thermo-regulatory centre in an adjacent part of the brain and it is the alteration in the function of the auto-nomic nervous system (that part of the nervous system over which we have no voluntary control) that leads to circulatory changes and the hot flushes and night sweats. Women who ex-perience an artificial menopause through surgery or medical treatment are much more likely to suffer such symptoms because the oestrogen withdrawal in their case is so much more abrupt.

Treatment

Conditions other than the menopause can cause night sweats and hot flushes, such as an overactive thyroid gland, untreated diabetes and allergic reactions. These are unusual, however. By and large, the circulation of blood in women who experience hot flushes and night sweats is much more sensitive to factors in our environment than normal, and it is this feeling of being out of control which is so loathed by menopausal women.

Self-help
- Try to identify any obvious trigger factors by making a mental note of them and later jotting them down.
- Alcohol is a potent dilator of blood vessels which will only make hot flushes worse, so cut down on alcohol as well as on spicy foods and garlic which can have similar effects.
- Cut down also on the number of hot drinks that you consume, especially caffeine-containing drinks like tea and coffee.
- Caffeine is also a nervous system, circulatory and cardiac stimulant as is nicotine, so avoid both.
- Especially avoid those hot drinks on an empty stomach and try to cut down on or quit smoking altogether.
- Keep as cool as possible because hot flushes and night sweats will always be worse when the ambient temperature is high. Avoid spending a lot of time outside in the heat of the day,

and keep temperatures inside the house at or below 19 degrees centigrade.

- During the day wear several thin layers of clothing rather than thick clothes so that you can shed layers easily without extra stress and embarrassment. In bed at night choose night-clothes and bedclothes made of natural fibres wherever possible and keep the window open to allow in some circulating air.
- Take helpful nutritional supplements such as vitamin E, evening primrose oil, magnesium and ginseng.
- Also try some aromatherapy, particularly concentrating on clary sage, geranium and lemon.
- Herbal infusions of sage may also help.
- Get a desk-top fan or small battery-operated fan to carry in your handbag. Also carry a handbag-sized water spray like the Evian spray.
- Keep your weight down because excess fatty tissue prevents your body radiating away heat which will make the hot flushes worse.
- If inconvenienced by a hot flush during the day, use a simple routine of slow deep breathing using an abbreviated 'quieting reflex' to inhibit the flush. This is simply a short de-stressing routine which prevents the release of chemicals, such as noradrenaline, which are the chemical messengers of stress. See box on page 50.

Another thing you can do with these symptoms is to get the best out of natural oestrogens, or phytoestrogens (see Chapter 11). Since only 10 per cent of Japanese women complain of hot flushes (compared with up to 80 per cent in the Western world) because of their higher dependence on phytoestrogens it seems logical to adopt their natural approach to this problem. Get into the habit too of exercising regularly. Exercise is probably the greatest stress buster of all, and it has a powerful effect in sharpening the reflexes required to control the opening up and closing down of the blood vessels in the skin which are responsible for hot flushes and night sweats. Exercise is also very beneficial in ironing out many of the

---

The Quieting Reflex

Close your eyes and identify what is irritating you. Say silently to yourself, 'A sharp mind and a relaxed body and I can deal with this.' Smile to yourself inwardly, without using any facial muscles. See yourself as a small child and imagine the child sitting on your lap now with your arms around her, protecting her. Now breathe in slowly to the count of four imagining the air coming in through the soles of your feet and slowly filling your abdomen, chest and then right to the top of your head. Now breathe out to the count of four. Imagine your breath passing downwards from the top of your head and out of your feet. Feel the goodness flowing through you. As you do this, relax your muscles and let your neck, jaw, shoulders and limbs go limp. Open your eyes now and carry on as before. With practice the quieting reflex can become so easy and automatic it can enable you to overcome any of the events during the day which make you irritable, frustrated and tense and which so often can trigger those annoying hot flushes.

---

mood swings which can arise as a result of hot flushes.

Positive thinking is important too in overcoming hot flushes and night sweats. According to Eastern religions and traditional medicine, these menopausal symptoms are regarded as a dramatic release of 'kundalini energy', a creative energy generated by the autonomic nervous system and endowing the woman with the power of healing as well as making her a source of wisdom and of peace keeping, the spiritual role of many post-menopausal women and matriarchs in many cultures. It can be helpful for some women to regard menopausal symptoms such as hot flushes in this way, so that instead of being something to be feared, the symptoms become a sign of that woman's individual spirit and regenerated energy coming to the fore. An alternative to the quietening reflex is visualisation exercises which can be taught by hypnotherapists, yoga teachers or relaxation therapists. Imagine sitting naked in a snow field and being rubbed all over with a moist towel full of ice cubes. This mental exercise alone, when practised regularly, can significantly bring about reflex cooling of the skin and the easing of symptoms.

Medical help

Undoubtedly, the most dramatically effective treatment for hot flushes is hormone replacement therapy which will improve symptoms in all cases where it is used appropriately. The effect of HRT is dose related, and women started off, as they usually are, on a low dose may need to be stepped up to a larger dose if their symptoms are not adequately controlled within two to three months. Since most women will cease having trouble-some hot flushes and night sweats within three years after the menopause, if HRT is being taken solely for the purpose of con-trolling these symptoms, it can be gradually discontinued later. To stop HRT suddenly is a mistake. There is now strong evidence that hot flushes are not caused by oestrogen deficiency in itself, but by oestrogen withdrawal. It is the falling level of oestrogen which triggers the symptoms. Younger women who go through a very early menopause often have no experience of hot flushes at all as their body and their circulation has never become 'sensitised' to high levels of oestrogen. Such women are often prescribed HRT because of their premature meno-pause and only ever experience hot flushes when the HRT is subsequently withdrawn, if that withdrawal is too sudden. So the underlying message is that HRT can be dramatically effec-tive but if it is discontinued in the future, this should only be done so on a gradual basis to avoid the problem of rebound symptoms. Progestogens such as medroxyprogestogerone acetate or megestrol acetate are also useful in controlling hot flushes, with a reduction of about 70 per cent with a dose of 20mg twice a day of megestrol. For those women for whom HRT is not suitable as a treatment, progestogens therefore are a good alternative. If you are unhappy with the idea of taking hormone replacement therapy in any shape or form there are a number of other medications which you might wish to discuss with your doctor. These include clonidine and propranolol, both of which can control changes in the calibre of blood vessels which is the mechanism whereby the symptom of flushing comes about.

IRREGULAR PERIODS

During the perimenopause, irregular bleeding is the symptom which bothers women more than anything else. We know that up to 80 per cent of menopausal women in Westernised countries suffer from hot flushes and night sweats and about 20 per cent seek medical help to alleviate them. But a greater proportion of women seek help for irregular bleeding which can consist of lighter periods, heavier periods, more frequent periods or periods which last longer or shorter than normal. Irregular menstrual bleeding is one of the first signs of falling oestrogen levels in the perimenopausal woman, and irregular bleeding can occur at any time from the late thirties onwards, although the commonest age at which these symptoms are reported is in the early forties onwards, preceding the menopause itself by anything from two to eight years.

Many doctors assume that irregular periods are due to the gradual onset of the menopause, but it is worth considering other causes of disturbed bleeding patterns which should never be ignored. Any dramatic weight loss can cause periods to stop as can excessive vigorous exercise. Physical and emotional upsets can disturb the body's hormone balance, and pregnancy should never be ignored as a possible cause of absent periods. Breast-feeding will inhibit bleeding and an early miscarriage is a possible cause of heavier or delayed bleeding and is something that should always be considered if contraception is not being used. In addition, disorders of the uterus itself, such as endometriosis, fibroids or a pre-cancerous build up of cells in the lining of the cavity of the uterus, so called endometrial hyperplasia, can all result in abnormal patterns of vaginal bleeding. A cervical erosion (softening of the neck of the womb) or cancer of the cervix are other possibilities, making regular cervical smears even more important. Inter-uterine contraceptive devices or coils, which many women in their forties rely on for contraception, are well known for increasing menstrual loss at period time or causing spotting between periods in some women. A list of these causes of abnormal bleeding is summarised in the box:

Causes of abnormal vaginal bleeding

1. Vigorous exercise
2. Dramatic weight loss
3. Eating disorders
4. Emotional upsets
5. Stress
6. Pregnancy
7. Breast-feeding
8. Miscarriage
9. Endometriosis, fibroids, endometrial hyperplasia
10. Cervical erosion
11. Cervical cancer
12. Intra-uterine contraceptive device
13. Menopause
14. Polyps
15. Herbals

Usually the first sign that you are approaching your menopause are periods which are more frequent, say every 21 days. The length of your cycle will shorten because the first half of your cycle, when follicle stimulating hormone is released, becomes shorter. Consequently, the second half of the cycle is moved forward and bleeding occurs earlier. Many women may be surprised by these more frequent periods because they expected less frequent periods if anything as it is commonly known that nearer to the menopause the periods become longer and longer apart and then stop altogether. But of course not all women experience more frequent periods. Some will have periods at the expected time but much heavier ones. We know that a third of women aged 45 to 50 have menstrual cycles where ovulation is missed altogether, and because ovulation is missed there is no corpus luteum or follicle sac left behind in the ovary, consequently no progesterone is produced to balance the effect of oestrogen in thickening the womb lining. Since the thickening increases in this exaggerated way, when the lining of the womb *is* finally shed, it may well be heavier and more prolonged.

Generally speaking, women have irregular periods for about four years before the periods finally stop altogether. Ten per cent of women will stop their periods quite dramatically, but others will be inconvenienced by irregular periods for five or six years. Even women who believe they have already gone through their menopause because they have stopped menstruating for over a year, may menstruate again on one or two occasions. These women and any woman who experiences very heavy bleeding (flooding) on a regular basis must see their doctor to rule out any of the other causes of these symptoms, which may sometimes prove to be unrelated to the menopause. Any bleeding which occurs between periods, after love-making or following the menopause must always be reported to the doctor for routine investigation of other possible causes. A menstrual diary is extremely helpful when discussing the menopause with a doctor and on it should be recorded the day of the menstrual cycle, when and how much bleeding occurs, and the presence of any physical or emotional symptoms as well. An example of a menstrual diary can be seen in Figure 9.

Treatment

Self-help
As soon as your periods become irregular or heavy, it is always worth taking extra iron and B group vitamins, along with vitamin C to absorb the iron more efficiently, to offset the possibility of anaemia. Increasing your dietary intake of phyto-estrogens is also useful as these can help to balance out regular production of oestrogen by the body in the perimenopause. It will become necessary to use heavier sanitary protection, perhaps using super-plus absorbency tampons and pads, and because periods can occur more frequently and often unexpectedly, a constant supply should always be kept on hand.

Medical help
In terms of treatment much depends on the severity of your symptoms, the impact they are having on your lifestyle and of course on your daily commitments in terms of home life and career. Amongst the various treatments available, medical solutions

Date of first day of your period			
Day	Bleeding	Physical	Emotional
1			
2			
3			
4			
5			
6			
7			
8			
9			
10			
11			
12			
13			
14			
15			
16			
17			
18			
19			
20			
21			
22			
23			
24			
25			
26			
27			
28			
29			
30			
31			

Day 1 is traditionally so-called as it represents the first day of your period.

Bleeding symptoms: record the letter S for spotting or P for period.

Physical symptoms: record H for headache, SP for spots, BP for back pain, AP for abdominal pain or BR for tender breasts.

Emotional symptoms: record I for irritable, T for tense, C for crying or N for normal.

Figure 9 **Menstrual diary**

and various forms of surgery are available. Since menstrual problems are often temporary or short lived during the perimenopause, and because such symptoms can often be made worse by stress, it makes sense to experiment with medical treatments first rather than considering any form of more drastic surgery. Surgery at any rate is only likely to offer benefits for a few years at the most since after the menopause has finished the problem of bleeding finishes altogether anyway.

Non-hormonal treatments

These can be taken during the period itself to relieve symptoms such as cramps or heavy blood loss.

Mefanamic acid (Ponstan) is probably the best known of a group of medicines called prostaglandin inhibitors, prostaglandin being the chemical responsible within the lining of the womb for cramps and heavy bleeding. The effect of medicines like mefanamic acid is only mild, however, reducing blood loss by 30–40 per cent at most, which can still prove inadequate if the vaginal loss is very heavy.

Ibuprofen which can be bought over the counter in pharmacies belongs to the same group of medicines as mefanamic acid and can be good for easing menstrual cramps, although its role in reducing heavy bleeding has yet to be fully evaluated.

Another non-hormonal treatment for irregular periods is tranexamic acid (Cyclokapron) which inhibits excessive blood loss by helping the blood to clot more effectively within the lining of the womb. It is only available on prescription, but it is capable of reducing menstrual flow by up to 50 per cent. It does not, however, relieve period cramps. It is taken as soon as heavy bleeding begins and can be taken simultaneously with a painkiller. It is usually taken in two tablets three to four times a day during the days of heavier blood flow.

Hormone treatments

A more potent solution to menstrual problems at the perimenopause comes in the form of hormonal treatments. One of the commonest causes of irregular bleeding is the change in the levels of oestrogen produced by the ovaries in the build up to the menopause. Hormonal therapy is a logical way of correcting this. If ovulation fails to take place mid-cycle, as it often does in women from their mid-forties onwards, no corpus luteum is formed to produce progesterone. This is the hormone which helps to balance out the build up of the lining of the womb in response to oestrogen. Without this progesterone the uterine lining continues to thicken and build up, leading to heavier and sometimes delayed bleeding at period time.

Synthetic progesterone known as progestogen is therefore useful in balancing out the effect of the oestrogen, resulting in more regular and lighter periods. There are many different types of progestogen which can be taken in tablet form, and they are often given initially for, say, two to three weeks, to bring the bleeding under control, being prescribed thereafter for several months at critical pre-menstrual times to regulate the cycle. Minor side effects such as weight gain, nausea and bloating are sometimes reported, but serious side effects are unusual. It is possible to use natural progesterone, but because it is not efficient when taken orally nor as a cream applied to the skin, it really needs to be administered via the vagina or as a suppository placed in the rectum to be effective.

Hormone replacement therapy using oestrogen combined with progestogen is occasionally used to treat irregular bleeding in the perimenopause as it regulates the cycle, although it will not necessarily reduce heavy bleeding if the cycle is already regular. It can be prescribed for smokers regardless of age and even for some women who may have a history of heart disease as HRT consists of lower doses of 'natural' hormones compared with the oral contraceptive pill which contains artificial hormones at higher dosage. Women with heavy bleeding can be reassured that their periods are likely to become lighter with HRT and after the menopause there are certain special preparations of HRT which can be deliberately chosen to provide a bleed-free form of hormone replacement therapy.

Surgery

Sometimes, despite the best efforts of the patient and her doctor, medical treatments are insufficient to control symptoms and surgery may be the best overall choice. A gynaecologist may suggest a hysterectomy (removal of the uterus) but there are many different types of hysterectomy and there is also a good surgical alternative, which is less drastic and which does not involve the removal of the uterus at all, known as endometrial ablation.

Although hysterectomy is one of the commonest operations performed in Western countries, there is a growing concern that too many women may be having this operation and that a proportion of them have it despite having no significant or serious disease within the uterus. There is a growing feeling that the operation is carried out rather too routinely and sometimes unnecessarily, resulting in a number of women subsequently feeling psychologically harmed by the procedure because of the effect it might have had on their sexuality or their femininity. The vast majority of women, I'm glad to say, are entirely satisfied with the results of their surgery, but it is imperative that women understand all the various options to a surgical procedure for irregular periods associated with the menopause, and that they play a full part, in conjunction with their specialists, in coming to a decision with which they are entirely happy. If such informed consent is made, weighing up all the pros and cons of all the various options, there is very little chance that a woman will not be fully content with her treatment.

Endometrial ablation

Endometrial ablation is a surgical procedure whereby the lining of the womb is partially destroyed so that it ceases to bleed so much each month. It can be carried out in a number of ways, but the one principle these have in common is that they all avoid any need to make a surgical incision. The procedure is an example of 'minimally invasive' surgery. Gynaecologists will use the particular technique with which they are most familiar, and the success of the operation depends very much on the surgeon's experience. Some hospitals still can not offer this approach in treatment at all as no specialists in that hospital use the technique. Endometrial ablation is carried out mostly under general anaesthetic, and all of the procedures under its name are performed through the vagina, by passing instruments into the uterine cavity through the cervix. One type of procedure, known as trans-cervical resection of the endometrium (TCRE), removes a large proportion of the uterine lining in strips, employing a fine wire loop through which an electric current is passed (electrodiathermy). This heats up the muscle wall of the uterus at the same time as removing the lining, coagulating any blood vessels which would otherwise bleed heavily. The hollow chamber inside the uterus is continuously irrigated with fluid to wash out any blood and cellular debris. It also cools the tissues down. Other variations on the procedure use a roller-ball laser or radio-frequency waves, and even a balloon, as alternatives to electro-diathermy.

Amongst the other advantages of endometrial ablation is the fact that although the operations are carried out under general anaesthetic, they can be carried out on a day-case basis requiring just one overnight stay in hospital rather than the three to four days minimum required after hysterectomy. Return to work can often occur within three weeks, less than half the recovery time required after a full-blown hysterectomy. Possible complications can include unexpected bleeding and infection, and occasionally an accidental perforation of the uterus has been reported. No surgical method is completely free of risk but surveys show that only 2–6 per cent of endometrial ablation operations are followed by complications and this rate is lower than that of abdominal hysterectomy. The results of ablation treatment are that about 20 per cent of women have no menstrual bleeding at all two to three years after the procedure, and 50–60 per cent have reduced bleeding. On the down side, up to a quarter of women find that they experience no improvement and a very few can even report worsening of their symptoms. As time goes on, the menstrual flow can increase again, though if the procedure is conducted near to the menopause itself all such bleeding will cease within a short period of time anyway. Interestingly, despite the fact that 75 per cent of women treated with endometrial ablation are happy with the results of their operation (a higher number than those satisfied with medical treatments), the overall rate of hysterectomies being carried out in the country as a whole has not declined as a result. Any woman, therefore, who has tried medical treatments without success, who has completed her family, needs help with heavy bleeding and is not keen to have major surgery should seriously consider the option of endometrial ablation. It is not a suitable form of treatment for women who may wish to have children in the future, nor is it particularly suitable for women with very painful periods as these may not be relieved after ablation. In addition, endometrial ablation is not recommended for women with fibroids.

Hysterectomy

If, with the help of your specialist, you feel that a hysterectomy is the right form of treatment for you, you still need to decide on the type of procedure which will suit you best. The operation you have could involve the removal of all or just part of your uterus, and your ovaries may not need to be removed during the course of the operation. If the ovaries are to be removed, the reasons need to be fully explained and understood. In an abdominal hysterectomy your womb is removed through an abdominal incision located in the so-called 'bikini line'. The operation usually means a stay in hospital of somewhere between three and seven days and a recovery time varying anywhere between six and twelve weeks, depending on your general health, whether there are complications after surgery and also, of course, on your family and career commitments. A total abdominal hysterectomy is the operation which is most commonly performed and this involves removal of your uterus and its neck (cervix), leaving a scar at the top of the vagina as well as the one where the incision has been made on the abdomen. It will not usually include the removal of the ovaries unless there are particular reasons for this to be carried out.

Total hysterectomy means that cancer of the cervix can never develop in the future as the cervix is removed along with the uterus. Most women who have this treatment will therefore never have to have another cervical smear and any future concerns in this area can be avoided.

Some women nevertheless opt to have a sub-total hysterectomy whereby the neck of the womb is left in place. Provided the woman concerned has always had regular smears and they have always been negative, this is an option which is entirely reasonable if the woman herself requests it. Since the removal of the cervix is in any case one of the hardest parts of the operation, a sub-total hysterectomy is a simpler and safer operation. Some women also believe that the sexual stimulation of the cervix is important for sexual fulfilment and that therefore this kind of operation is advantageous, but research tells us that the majority of women do not experience any worsening in their love lives after removal of the cervix, so this perceived benefit may be exaggerated. None the less, it is a point meriting discussion between you and your doctor before surgery is carried out.

A vaginal hysterectomy is the procedure employed for treating a prolapsed uterus and it is less often used for a woman purely with irregular and/or heavy periods as it is technically more difficult and has the potential for more troublesome post-operative complications. During it, both the womb and the cervix are removed through an incision at the top of the vagina so no abdominal scar will be left. However, for the woman there may be less post-operative discomfort and recovery time is shorter than for abdominal hysterectomy. A woman can expect to be in hospital for an average of two to four days, followed by recovery in six to eight weeks. At the current time only about 12 per cent of hysterectomies in Britain are carried out by this method.

Preparation for a hysterectomy

The decision to undergo a hysterectomy is usually taken over a period of time when various medical treatments have already been tried. A hysterectomy carried out specifically for menstrual disorders would be one that does not need to be hurried. It is normal to feel concerned and apprehensive about a major operation, but only by being fully informed and adequately prepared can the anxiety be taken out of the procedure so you actually welcome the operation rather than regarding it with fear and dread. It is important to remember that it is not just you yourself on whom the operation has an impact but your partner, your family and possibly even your work colleagues. The bottom line is that if you decide to have a hysterectomy, it's essential to view it as the best possible solution for the particular problem in question, and all the above medical and surgical alternatives need to have been considered.

Another vital consideration is whether the gynaecologist is recommending that your ovaries be removed or not. This will depend on the circumstances and on the particular indication for the surgery, but it is a subject which simply must always be discussed since it has implications for menopausal symptoms afterwards.

Every woman should understand how long she can expect to be on the waiting list, and about the arrangements concerning her admission to hospital. You should find out how long you are likely to have to stay in hospital and how long recovery will take so that domestic and employment aspects may be considered. These days, on average, a woman will stay in hospital for three or four days after an abdominal hysterectomy, a much shorter time than was recommended some years ago. This is not because of bed shortages so much as the fact that with modern surgical treatment, nursing care and physiotherapy it has become clear that recovery takes place more efficiently when you return to your normal daily activities. Women having vaginal or other forms of surgery for menstrual irregularities may be home even more quickly. On the other hand, if a hysterectomy is being carried out for uterine or cervical cancer, the operation and recovery from it are liable to be more complicated.

So not all hysterectomies will have the same outcome, and you cannot necessarily assume that because somebody else you knew had a hysterectomy and had a certain post-operative regime, that it will be the same for you. At what time in the future you are likely to get back to work after your operation again depends on the type of operation and the kind of work you carry out. On average you are likely to be off for a minimum of six weeks, although an abdominal hysterectomy may require twelve weeks for full convalescence. Women who are overweight are normally advised to try to lose weight before the operation as not only does it make surgery easier for the surgeon, but it also reduces the risk of complications, from both the surgical procedure and the general anaesthetic used. It is a good idea to cut down on smoking or even give up altogether if possible to minimise the risk of chest infections after the operation. A smoker's cough is also likely to put more strain on the stitches and on the pelvic floor muscles following the procedure.

Some hospitals admit women having a hysterectomy the day before the operation so that you can be checked over, but other hospitals have a pre-admission clinic where you attend a week or so in advance so you can be examined routinely as an out-patient. Initial tests carried out as a matter of course include a chest x-ray, an ECG and blood tests which include those for cross-matching blood in case a transfusion may be required during the operation. Since some women may be anaemic as a result of heavy bleeding, these blood tests are particularly important because any anaemia would need to be corrected before surgery. Before signing the consent form, it is important to make sure the nature of the operation is completely understood, and that the decision regarding possible simultaneous removal of the ovaries has been made and agreed. The operation of hysterectomy is normally performed under a general anaesthetic which is administered after a 'pre-med' which helps the patient to relax and cuts down on fluid secretions in the respiratory passageways prior to the anaesthetic. The anaesthetist will have already asked you whether you have any prior health problems, such as allergy, and whether you take any regular medications.

VAGINAL DRYNESS

Vaginal dryness is an almost universal symptom after the menopause as oestrogen is vital in keeping the lining of the vagina
moist and well-lubricated. As oestrogen levels fall at and after
the menopause, blood flow is reduced within the vagina and
dryness becomes an extremely common problem. The vaginal
tissue becomes thinner and less elastic and what little secretions
are present have a higher pH (they are less acidic) than before
the menopause leading to a vulnerability to bacterial infection
and thrush. The more patriarchal medical experts amongst
Britain's gynaecologists refer to this problem as 'atrophic
vaginitis' or 'vaginal atrophy' or 'vulval dystrophy', whereby
pallor of the vaginal tissues, patches of broken blood vessels
called petechiae and absence of the folds of the vaginal lining
(rugae) are in evidence on examination. As a result of these
changes symptoms can occur such as burning, itching, pain and
bleeding. More frequent urinary infections or cystitis may also
occur as the urethra, the water pipe which runs along the front
wall of the vagina can become increasingly liable to trauma
during love-making. Because love-making is tender and uncomfortable, it is easy for you to lose confidence sexually and
consciously or unconsciously begin to avoid initiating sex with
your partner at all. This is true even if your sex drive, your libido,
is normal. With the best will in the world, even if you feel like
making love, if you know it is going to be uncomfortable or actually hurt, it can be a great turn off. Many a strong relationship
has foundered as a result of this simple truth. Interestingly,
research has shown that frequent sexual activity does still stimulate the production of vaginal moisture post-menopausally
although there will be less lubrication and it will take nearly five
times as long to produce as it did before the change. It would
appear that the same adage often used for men – 'if you don't
use it, you lose it' – may be equally applicable to women since
women who still enjoy frequent love-making post-menopausally
do not seem to suffer from vaginal dryness as much as those who
are less active.

Treatments

Self-help
Simple self-help measures that you can take include the avoidance of soaps and detergents which dry vaginal lubrication even more; so soaps, scented bath preparations like bubblebath and shower gels are all very worth while avoiding. You should wear loose cotton underclothes and avoid trousers which are tight around the crotch, and it is recommended that stockings are worn rather than nylon tights if possible. Many women even in their twenties and thirties suffer from lack of vaginal lubrication as constitutionally this is the way they are made. These same recommendations apply to them just as much before the menopause as afterwards. Another good self-help measure is the application of live natural yoghurt directly to the vagina as this increases acidity and reduces the risk of thrush infections otherwise known as candidiasis. The same acid-making bacilli, lacto-bacilli, can also be taken in tablet form and these are available from health-food shops. Other supplements worth trying include vitamin E preparations and oil of evening primrose. Herbalists suggest motherwort and chastetree taken internally, along with aloe vera, comfrey and calendula to be used externally. Not only are they useful in problems with vaginal dryness, but they may have some benefit in preventing recurrent vaginal and bladder infections too. Fifteen drops of tincture of motherwort in a glass of water several times a day can to some extent restore thickness to the vaginal lining and bring about more moisture. Chastetree berries can also be taken in tincture form, say 20 drops two or three times a day for similar effects. To relieve itching and to soften the vaginal tissues and the vulva, calendula officinalis is a useful cream, and so is comfrey (symphytum officinalis) for itching and burning. It can even be used as a lubricant instead of the more conventional ones, ideally used three times a day for three months initially to see whether any permanent effect has been achieved. Finally some women have found that the direct application of aloe vera juice in pure form can be helpful for atrophic

symptoms. It can simply be wiped on several times a day.

One of the features about vaginal dryness which puzzles doctors, is that there seems to be little correlation between the findings during close examination and the symptoms. Some women have symptoms with very little change visible, whereas other women have no symptoms when fairly obvious physical changes have occurred. For this reason, self-help measures are well worth trying by any woman suffering from vaginal dryness, before recourse to more powerful treatments. Another important tip for women suffering from discomfort during intercourse is to make sure that she and her partner enjoy extended foreplay prior to love-making. Aromatherapy massage in particular can be very relaxing and conducive to fulfilling romance; it involves just a few drops of a good aromatherapy oil mixed with almond oil and these can be bought over the counter at any pharmacy. Massage can be carried out prior to love-making on a mutual basis. There is no reason why a woman should not be enjoying a fulfilling sex life if she wants one and it is important that she takes measures to preserve that sex life by all reasonable means possible.

Medical help
Additional help can be found at pharmacies and in doctors' surgeries. Sometimes extra lubrication may be all that is required. The water-based KY jelly is a popular solution and so is polycarbophil (Replens) which can be used by way of an applicator just three times a week to increase lubrication, increase vaginal acidity and dispense with the usual symptoms of atrophy. Whereas KY jelly is generally used immediately prior to intercourse when it takes place, Replens may be used at any time every other day. Hormonal therapies can be used in natural or pharmaceutical form. Phytoestrogens, the ones which are derived from plant material, are well worth trying and may have an adequate effect on vaginal secretions to ease symptoms. However, synthetic hormone replacement therapy on prescription is more dramatically effective for this potentially distressing consequence of the menopause. HRT given orally, in implant

form, by injection or through skin patches will almost always result in better moisturisation and thickening of the vaginal lining. But sometimes additional HRT in vaginal cream form may be necessary. Women whose only menopausal symptom is vaginal dryness should be recommended vaginal cream only in the first instance as this may be sufficient, but for women who are taking oral HRT in small dosage and who still get symptoms, it is probably better to add a vaginal cream rather than to increase the dose of their tablets. Another vaginal moisturiser of non-hormonal type is Senselle. Along with KY Jelly and Replens, this is available from most high-street chemists or can be ordered.

Treatments for vaginal dryness

Avoid scented soaps and bubblebath.
Wear loose cotton underclothes.
Wear stockings rather than tights.
Apply live yoghurt, comfrey or calendula cream, aloe vera juice or herbal tinctures.
Take vitamin E, oil of evening primrose, motherwort and chastetree.
Try aromatherapy massage as part of foreplay.
Take more phytoestrogens in your diet.
Try KY jelly, Replens or other vaginal lubricant.
Ask about HRT as vaginal cream or other forms.

PUTTING ON WEIGHT

There is no doubt that many women seem to put on weight at and around the time of the menopause although many of them unfairly blame this weight gain on HRT if it is prescribed. But contrary to popular opinion, there is evidence that HRT actually reduces weight gain at this time and there are a number of reasons why the menopause itself can be responsible.

We know that there is already an increasing prevalence of obesity in Britain as people are eating more and taking less exercise. At the time of the menopause there are additional reasons why your weight may increase. Although not all women become heavier the majority do, partly because of changes in lifestyle and partly because the body's ability to burn up calories (the 'basal metabolic rate') naturally declines. Lifestyle changes mean that your activities can become more sedentary and perhaps joint and muscular aches and pains may increasingly discourage physical exertion. In addition, fear of urinary leakage due to stress incontinence, or fear of overdoing it after a surgical operation like a hysterectomy can lead to decreased physical activity. But even if you take the same amount of exercise and eat the same diet you may still put on weight because your metabolic rate naturally slows by as much as 12 per cent by your mid-forties compared with 20 years earlier, which means that your body needs fewer calories to produce the same amount of energy. Another factor leading to weight gain is water retention which can occur in the aftermath of hormonal fluctuation at this time. This may also occur as a short-lived side effect of HRT if it is prescribed.

One of the major changes of the menopause is that falling levels of oestrogen mean that you begin to store any excess weight in a different pattern of distribution around your body. Instead of putting on weight around the traditional problem areas, such as the breasts, hips and thighs, the extra fatty tissue is laid down in the abdominal area just as it is in men. This in turn leads to loss of the normal pre-menopausal female figure, so post-menopausally you become less pear-shaped and more apple-shaped. This change in shape is interesting from a medical perspective because just as apple-shaped men with a high waist to hip measurement are more likely to run risks of coronary heart disease, strokes, high blood pressure, high cholesterol levels, gall stones and diabetes, so are women after the menopause as they adopt a similar figure. So, quite apart from reasons of wanting to feel good about yourself, any post-menopausal woman should make all reasonable attempts to keep her weight to within normal limits for health reasons. The best measurement of weight is the Body Mass Index or BMI.

BODY MASS INDEX READY RECKONER

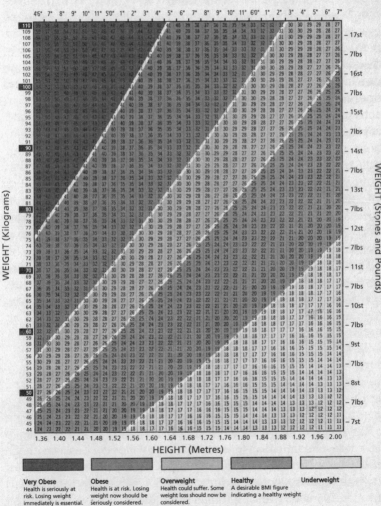

HEIGHT (Feet and Inches)

WEIGHT (Kilograms)

WEIGHT (Stones and Pounds)

HEIGHT (Metres)

Very Obese
Health is seriously at
risk. Losing weight
immediately is essential.

Obese
Health is at risk. Losing
weight now should be
seriously considered.

Overweight
Health could suffer. Some
weight loss should now be
considered.

Healthy
A desirable BMI figure
indicating a healthy weight

Underweight

© Servier Laboratories Limited 1991

This is the weight in kilograms divided by the height in metres squared:

$$BMI = \text{weight (kilos) divided by height (metres)}^2$$

See the Body Mass Index Ready Reckoner, which shows height in metres against weight in kilos, and BMI levels. Imperial measurements are also given.

Women with a BMI between 20 and 25 are in the right weight range for their height but about 30 per cent of UK women are overweight, with a BMI between 25 and 30, and over 15 per cent are obese, with a BMI of more than 30.

Treatment

Self-help

A healthy lifestyle with moderate amounts of a balanced variety of foods plus adequate exercise is the ideal way to avoid putting on weight at the menopause. Calorie intake needs to be adjusted according to normal daily levels of activity. An office worker or someone whose career involves sitting at a desk, who is unable to take much exercise, clearly needs less of a calorie intake than someone who exercises daily, who indulges in heavy duty gardening or is an agricultural worker. Here are some essential tips for keeping weight down:

1. Stick to a sensible diet. Fruit and vegetables provide energy, have an extremely low fat content, are filling and satisfying, and help also with menopausally related conditions such as constipation and irritable bowel syndrome. Choose low-fat varieties of spreads and dairy products such as milk and cheeses, and go for crème-fraîche rather than cream on desserts. Avoid all fried foods and grill the very leanest cuts of meat whenever possible.
2. Join a weight-control club to share ideas and become motivated by others.
3. Try to find priority time for regular aerobic exercise at least three times a week. This will improve muscle tone and make you look and feel better even if your weight remains the same.

4. Keep a food diary which records when, where and what is eaten and correlate it to how you feel. Are you bored, are you fed up, for example?

5. Identify any situations which tend to encourage you to eat when you are not really hungry. For instance, if the office coffee break always results in you eating a chocolate bar try to avoid going there and choose an alternative place for a break. Try to avoid eating between meals. If you do feel peckish snack on healthy foodstuffs such as carrots or celery and make each proper meal an occasion where you take your time and eat slowly, savouring your food as you do.

6. Avoid shopping when you are hungry and only shop from a pre-prepared list.

7. Avoid comfort eating. If you know you tend to eat as a form of comfort, when you are stressed or upset, find alternative ways to relax such as listening to soothing music, enjoying some aromatherapy, taking a hot bath or enjoying exercise.

8. Avoid temptation. Eat normal-sized portions of normal-sized servings of foods and do not cook more than you need. Resist finishing off any left-overs and sampling any cooking when it is being prepared. Get into the habit of waiting for twenty-five to thirty minutes after your main course before tucking into those high calorie desserts as it takes your body about half an hour for blood sugar levels to increase after eating and abolish hunger pains.

9. Increase your intake of phytoestrogens (see Chapter 11). Increase your intake of soya milk or other soya products. Consider supplements such as red clover, alfalfa and vervain. The vegetables in your staple diet should include plenty of legumes, with chick peas, lentils, mung beans and aduki beans being amongst those that contain substantial levels of all the four major isoflavones which counteract the effect of diminishing oestrogen levels within the body.

Medical help

So what is the role of hormone replacement therapy in dealing with or contributing to menopausal weight gain?

Many women blame HRT for weight gain after the menopause

but for all the reasons discussed above weight gain will occur naturally at the menopause anyway. In fact there is now broad agreement amongst doctors and scientists that HRT in the long term prevents an increase in body weight and in skin fold thickness and that it reduces the tendency for women to redistribute fatty tissue around the abdominal region. Clinical research has shown that body weight and the BMI is reduced in women who take HRT, especially in women who are not obese before they start taking it. A very recent article in the *Journal of Endocrinology* (devoted to the study of the glandular and hormonal system) showed significant reductions in the accumulation of fat around the torso region in women when they took HRT for five years compared to similar numbers of women who did not take HRT. They confirmed that the effect of HRT was especially significant in women who were not overweight prior to treatment as opposed to women who were, attributing this observed difference to altered levels of insulin and free fatty acids in those women who were overweight, which in turn could reduce the effect of the prescribed oestrogen. Whilst HRT should not be used purely to control any possible weight gain in menopausal women without any other symptoms, there are good grounds for reassurance in women for whom HRT is suggested and who have been misguided by the myth that HRT is always responsible for weight gain. This is certainly a subject worth discussing more fully with your doctor.

URINARY PROBLEMS

Urinary problems are very common after the menopause, affecting more than 50 per cent of women at some time in their post-menopausal lives. They are frequently viewed as one of the most humiliating of all symptoms relating to the change and it is very clear that many women suffer in silence, being too embarrassed to mention these kind of symptoms to their doctors at all. The most common symptoms include frequency, which is the constant desire to visit the loo to empty the bladder; urgency, which is the immediate and urgent need to pass urine, and which if not obeyed often results in wetting; and finally stress incontinence, when laughing, coughing, sneezing, exercise or even sexual activity can lead to urinary leakage. There is also an increased tendency after the menopause for frequent bladder infections to take place, resulting in cystitis. Medically the underlying causes of these problems include weakening of the special triangle at the neck of the bladder which is less able to control urinary flow. There is also a decreased sensitivity of the nerves at the bladder neck as well as thinning of the mucosa, the delicate lining in the water pipe (urethra) itself. Overall, bladder weakness affects three million people of all ages in Britain today with two out of five women developing bladder problems at some stage. Most women with bladder weakness problems do not leak large quantities all at once but maybe just a few drops or small gushes of urine. Stress incontinence is caused by weakness in the pelvic floor muscles which support the bladder outlet and which become stretched and weakened during childbirth. Being overweight also puts extra strain on these pelvic floor muscles and can contribute therefore to symptoms. In addition, certain medications, constipation and even infections can make any minor bladder weakness worse. After the menopause, when the circulating levels of oestrogen begin to fall, there is a relative acceleration in the degenerative processes which in turn leads to less support for the vagina and bladder outlet. At the same time, because of lowered oestrogen levels, the normal acidity of the vagina is reduced, leading to a change in the normal bacterial flora and an increase in the number of gram-negative organisms such as E. Coli, thus making a likelihood of bacterial cystitis very real. Such organisms can easily ascend from the vaginal area to the bladder to cause recurrent infection.

Treatments

Self-help
It is important to try to keep the bladder as healthy as possible through simple self-help measures.

- Drink plenty of fluid – say three to four pints every day and more if necessary in hot weather or if you have been exercising. This makes the kidneys filter more urine from the blood, diluting any germs that may be present in the urinary system and flushing out any micro-organisms that may otherwise tend to ascend upwards towards the bladder and kidneys.
- Still water is the best drink of all as too much alcohol and caffeine-containing drinks like tea, coffee and many fizzy drinks can cause irritation and bring about the onset of symptoms in their own right.
- Try to relax, instead of straining to empty the bladder. It is always best to sit on the toilet seat rather than hovering above it for fear that it may not be absolutely clean.
- Bladder training, and re-training if necessary, is also important. Try not to hold back for too long when you feel the need to empty the bladder, on the other hand try not to run to the loo every five minutes just in case you might not be able to get to a loo easily within the next half an hour. This merely serves to make the bladder gradually contract so that any small volume within it increases the sensation of fullness and the need to go.
- Try also to keep bowel movements regular as a loaded colon can press upon the bladder leading to frequency and other problems.
- Frequent urinary infections can sometimes be reduced by taking herbal supplements such as cranberry juice, which alters the acidity of the urine favourably and inhibits the growth of micro-organisms. Similar preparations can be purchased over the counter at the chemist such as potassium citrate and other powders that may be dissolved in water to achieve much the same effect as natural cranberry juice.
- Safe discreet protection is also now available, allowing women to be social and active even when experiencing bladder problems regularly. Women will have got used to using panty-liners or sanitary towels for menstruation before the menopause but there is a major difference between the

products made for urinary incontinence and those made for menstruation. Newer products like Tena-Lady Pads are able to absorb large amounts of urine quickly and keep it locked inside the pad. Modern products are also specially designed to counteract any unpleasant odour and the lower pH contributes to healthier skin. The pads are comfortably shaped and contoured to fit the body so they are flexible, comfortable and discreet. They also come in different sizes to provide for women of different shapes and different needs.

- It is also well worth strengthening the pelvic floor muscles by carrying out Kegel exercises on a daily basis. These are successful for 10–25 per cent of women. See box on page 76.

Medical help
For older women with any degree of prolapse of the womb and looseness of the vaginal walls, ring pessaries may be an effective solution. These are firm PVC rings that are inserted high up into the vagina (behind the pubic bone and into the vault of the vagina behind the cervix) to hold up and support the vaginal tissues, preventing the womb from descending. They are very useful in controlling urinary incontinence as a result of an unsupported urethra but they are really only suitable for older women.

The other technique to help strengthen pelvic floor muscles is the use of a series of weighted vaginal cones. Initially only light weights are held within the vagina until control is achieved, leading on later to heavier weights as the muscles become stronger. Sets of these vaginal weighted cones can be purchased or even borrowed from local hospital physiotherapy departments.

When these measures fail further help from the medical profession can be very useful. For severe frequency, urgency and stress incontinence, some of the newer medicines which act to stabilise the muscular wall of the bladder can be very useful in controlling symptoms. Many of these are 'anti-cholinergic' in action, blocking the effect of nervous stimulation of the bladder wall. Such medicines as propiverine are available in tablet form,

How to perform Kegel exercises

The techniques can be learnt once an understanding of the right muscle groups has been obtained. To do this sit, stand or lie down. Without tensing the muscles of the abdomen, buttocks or legs, internally tighten the ring of muscle around the back passage by imagining that you were trying to control the passing of the bowel motion. That helps to identify the back part of the pelvic floor. Next time you are emptying the bladder try to stop the flow of urine in mid-stream and then re-start it. This will enable you to become aware of the front muscles of the pelvic floor. Initially it may only be possible to slow down the stream rather than stop it altogether but as the muscles become stronger through the exercises, you will be able to stop the flow completely. This exercise does not need to be repeated each time you go to the toilet, only once a day at the most. Having found the pelvic floor muscles, carry out exercises working back to front and tightening the muscles while counting to four slowly, then releasing them. Attempt to do this every quarter of an hour for the next three months if possible. As the muscles become stronger and more under your control you will find that it is possible to do these exercises anywhere anytime. Sitting in the chair at the office, watching television at home, preparing food in the kitchen or even standing in the supermarket checkout queue. Nobody will know what you are up to. After doing this for two to three weeks you should be aware of voluntary closing down of the back and front passages and a drawing up of the pelvic floor in front. Remember not to allow the leg, tummy or buttock muscles to tense as it is unlikely that the right pelvic muscles will be used otherwise. Pelvic floor muscles are inside the body, not on the outside.

the recommended dose being one 15mg tablet two or three times a day.

As for hormone replacement therapy, the jury is still out to some extent on how useful this may be in treating urinary problems. In one study where vaginal oestriol cream was used for women who had recurrent infection, a good response was obtained in many cases. This is because oestrogen can delay many of the degenerative processes which lead to infection in the first place. It also increases vaginal acidity once again making the growth of troublesome organisms more unlikely. In terms of stress and urge incontinence, the results of using HRT are more mixed. Overall, however, there seems to be a small beneficial effect in helping the symptoms of urinary incontinence through using HRT and if oral or patch forms in normal dosage do not produce an adequate effect, oestrogen in the form of vaginal cream, vaginal tablets or vaginal rings are preferable as an addition to the small dose rather than the other option of increasing the dose of the tablets or patches. Vagifem is available in Britain, it is an oestrogen vaginal tablet and is used in a dose of one tablet inserted vaginally twice a week. An oestrogen ring known as Estring is a silicone elastima ring with a core containing two milligrams of oestradiol and this is inserted and replaced every ninety days. Ovestin is an oestrogen cream applied vaginally twice weekly.

Finally, for women with any degree of prolapse in whom stress incontinence is seriously affecting their quality of life, surgery either to tighten the pelvic floor muscles once again or to remove the womb completely through vaginal hysterectomy may be the best and most definitive solution to improving symptoms. Medical treatments for incontinence are summarised in the box below:

Medical treatments for incontinence

Ring pessaries
Weighted vaginal cones
Anti-cholinergic medication
HRT in vaginal tablet, cream, ring or other form
Surgery

DRY SKIN AND WRINKLES

During the peri-menopause and thereafter the skin becomes progressively thinner as it loses collagen, the scaffolding material which supports it. Elastic fibres are also reduced in number with the result that wrinkles, fine lines, crow's feet and lipstick lines all begin to become more obvious. Many of these changes come about as a result of accumulated exposure to ultra-violet light from the sun, and smoking also undoubtedly accelerates the ageing process within the skin. Stress is another factor which can lead to tension in the muscles beneath the facial skin, and to frowning which only encourages wrinkles. Hot baths, dehydration as a result of living or working in centrally heated offices without adequate ventilation, and not drinking enough fluid are other possible factors.

At the menopause relative oestrogen deficiency is very strongly thought to be an important factor in dry skin and wrinkles, and in a recent and very large scientific study involving some 4,000 post-menopausal women, those who took hormone replacement therapy had fewer wrinkles and less dry skin with a difference of some 25–30 per cent of benefit over those women who did not take HRT. This points very strongly towards an oestrogenic benefit. Since one of the greatest compliments a woman over 40 can ever be paid is to be told that she looks ten years younger than she really is, solutions for dry skin and wrinkles are highly sought after. Ask most women and they will tell you that the appearance of their skin has an important part to play, not only in their self-esteem, but in their social life and even their career prospects. Many feel that the appearance of their skin is as important as acne is for teenagers or male pattern baldness is for men. So much so that British women spend more than £350 million a year on skin care products of which more than £100 million is spent on moisturisers alone. These make all sorts of claims including the prevention, slowing down and repair of ageing skin, although most of them offer more hope than real measurable effect. There are of course products which protect and nourish the skin to some extent, improving the appearance of the skin, and certainly dry skin will tend to wrinkle earlier than oily skin. Many women genetically have drier skin than others, in which case they will tend to have associated problems such as eczema or psoriasis, whereas other women, particularly with black skin, will have oilier skin in which case acne is the equivalent associated problem. Unfortunately dry skin, wrinkles and even acne can become more prominent at the menopause. Acne can occur as a result of waning oestrogen levels which allow the small amounts of testosterone in a woman's body to stimulate sebum (oil) production in the skin, leading to the characteristic signs of acne. Dry skin and wrinkles become more obvious as a result of falling oestrogen levels for reasons already discussed.

Treatment

Self-help
There is much a menopausal woman can do to minimise detrimental effects on her skin.

- Avoiding smoking is vital because just ten cigarettes a day for two years can double the number of premature wrinkles according to American research. Smoking releases harmful free radicals in the body, depletes vitamin C and reduces the supply of oxygen to cells. It weakens collagen within the skin and breaks up elastic fibres, leading to sagging and wrinkling. Smokers often have the same number of wrinkles at the age of 40 as non-smokers have at the age of 60, with particularly prominent lines around the eyes and lips.
- Too much alcohol is also bad for the skin as excess amounts dehydrate the body depriving cells of essential moisture and leading to premature ageing. Drinking too reduces vital nutrients such as vitamins A, B and C, magnesium, zinc and essential fatty acids.
- These important nutrients can also be reduced by a high caffeine intake, so too much coffee, tea and cola-based fizzy drink and chocolate are worth avoiding as well. One hypothesis explaining why excess coffee might be harmful to the skin involves a certain ingredient called benzoic acid. This can only be excreted by the kidneys when it has been converted into hippuric acid by an amino acid called glycine. Since this

amino acid is found in collagen as well as in the liver, the body diverts it from skin collagen in order to get rid of benzoic acid toxins so depleting levels in the skin. How significant this effect might be remains to be seen.

- Reducing the amount of saturated animal fat in the diet, going easy on salt and keeping refined sugar intake to modest amounts is also likely to have huge benefits for the skin.
- A generally sensible diet which avoids both over-eating and yoyo dieting is also likely to be conducive to a satisfactory dermatological appearance.
- Saturated fats should be eaten in moderation as they can contribute to heart disease over the years as well as causing a spotty sallow-looking skin. Cut down on full fat dairy products and instead choose polyunsaturated and mono-unsaturated fats derived predominantly from vegetables and plants. Virgin olive oil, sunflower oil, walnut and sesame oil are all preferable to saturated fats and essential fatty acids and fish oils are vital in keeping skin cells healthy.
- The most important thing of all, however, to keep the skin healthy and attractive is to avoid excessive exposure to sunlight, something which involves the regular application of sunscreen whenever appropriate. This measure is also likely to cut down on irregular skin pigmentation and the development of unsightly skin tags around the neck and chest area.
- Since stress is a factor in the development of premature ageing of the skin adequate rest and relaxation is useful too. An effective skin care routine can certainly help. For most skins an oil-based cleanser is preferable, used morning and evening. Moisturisers maintain water in the stratum corneum, the outer layer of the skin, and it does not really matter which type is used provided it feels comfortable. Most commercially available perfumed soaps contain detergents which leech out natural oil from the skin and make it drier. Choose only non-drying soaps such as Simple Soap or even Aqueous Cream, available over the counter at the chemist, or choose a soap with a slightly acidic pH akin to normal skin's natural protective acidity. A water spray or spray-on tonic is

also helpful for keeping up the skin's moisture level throughout the day, particularly if you work in a dry environment. Weekly exfoliation is also beneficial to improve the texture of the skin as it removes dead skin cells that accumulate and give the skin a dull dry and flaky appearance.

- Supplements worth considering include all the antioxidant vitamins, particularly vitamins A, C and E, along with evening primrose oil and borage oil, both of which contain high levels of gammalinolenic acid (GLA), an essential fatty acid known to increase moisture levels in skin cells.
- In addition, herbs such as echinacea and dong quai are thought by herbalists to have a complementary effect.
- Never forget to take plenty of pure filtered water or bottled mineral water to prevent dehydration and to help filter out potentially harmful toxins from the body.

Medical help

From the medical point of view, menopausal women with particularly troublesome dry skin can be prescribed moisturising products such as Aveeno. This is a colloidal oatmeal product which can be added directly to the bath water or applied direct to the skin when showering and is also available in cream form. Ten per cent urea creams and other emulsifying ointments are prescribable if necessary. There is also a steroid-free emollient cream available over the counter in chemists which is hypoallergenic, preservative-free and useful not just for dry skin but for other dry itchy skin conditions such as eczema and psoriasis. It contains functional ingredients such as phytosterols, borage oil, aloe vera, zinc oxide and vitamin E amongst others.

An important contributory factor producing lines and wrinkles is loss of muscle tone, which occurs during the menopause particularly in the facial area, the only area of the body where skin is actually attached to underlying muscles. Many women find that these facial muscles can be toned up through specific exercises in much the same way that the pelvic floor muscles can be tightened, so learning where the muscles are and how they work is the first step. These are the basic facial exercises.

To strengthen the muscles around the jaw, mouth and cheeks, make vowel sounds A E I O U in a slow but exaggerated fashion opening the mouth as wide as possible and repeating it five times.

For the forehead, chin and cheek muscles hold down the skin above the eyebrows with the ends of your index fingers then try to push the eyebrows up and out with your brow muscles. Hold this for a count of five and repeat it five times.

For the mouth, nose and cheeks place the little fingers inside the corner of the mouth either side, pull the fingers outwards towards the sides and resist this pull with your mouth muscles. Again hold this for a count of five and repeat five times.

Finally, to strengthen the muscles which define the contours of the cheekbones, put the middle finger on top of your index finger and place both fingers just inside the mouth. By sucking inwards hard and holding for the count of five these muscles can be strengthened over the course of time. This exercise should be repeated up to ten times.

Hormone replacement therapy is likely to be beneficial to skin changes occurring at the menopause as studies suggest that women who take it may have fewer wrinkles and less dry skin than women who do not. It can make a difference of up to 25–30 per cent. See Chapter 13 (benefits of HRT). Few doctors would be willing to prescribe HRT purely to enhance the look of your skin but if other menopausal changes are causing symptoms, this benefit may still be the final factor if you are making up your mind about whether you want to take it or not.

Surgery
Most women accept that a certain amount of ageing is natural and inevitable. Despite such attitudes, increasing numbers of women feel they would like to do something about the way they look and turn to cosmetic surgery to provide the answers. Finding out all about what cosmetic surgery can and cannot do, how much it might cost and what is involved is then essential in obtaining the required result. Always ask your GP first about the treatment you might be contemplating and if necessary he or

she can refer you to a personally recommended surgeon. When seeing a cosmetic or aesthetic surgeon, ask to speak to other women who have been treated by them, and seek more than one opinion before making your final choice.

If you want to change your appearance because you want to feel good about yourself and improve your self-esteem that is fine but you should never undergo surgery purely because this is what your partner wants. You should understand that there is no guarantee of success.

When considering surgical cosmetic treatments the following options are normally available.

Chemical peels: First of all there are chemical peels which use high concentrations of alphahydroxyacids (AHAs), trichloro-aceticacid (TCA) or phenol to literally peel off the outer layers of skin revealing younger and smoother skin beneath. In achieving this, some of the fine lines and wrinkles are eradicated at the same time. Skin will appear red and slightly crusty after the peel for some two or three weeks after which healing takes place completely revealing the softer younger-looking skin. The technique is quite uncomfortable and must be carried out by a competent and experienced surgeon otherwise scarring, infection or patchy-looking skin are more likely to occur.

Dermabrasion: This is a similar technique but it removes the outer layers of the skin using an instrument resembling a mechanical sander. Dermabrasion is also used to remove many types of skin blemish including acne pits, scars and chicken pox dimples as well as brown patches and superficial fine lines. It is ideal for treating the pucker marks which develop around the lips causing lipstick to 'bleed'. Dermabrasion, like chemical peels, encourages the skin to reconstruct itself and promotes the production of collagen, the skin's scaffolding. Neither technique, however, has any lasting effect on sagging skin or on the nose-to-mouth grooves which may be prominent. The results depend on exactly how deeply the skin has been penetrated and, just as in chemical peeling, enlarged pores, discolouration and bleaching of the treated area which leaves a tide mark at the edges, can sometimes occur. The bleaching effect occurs because melanocytes, the cells which produce the brown pigment melanin that gives skin its colour and makes it turn brown in the sun, can be removed if the skin is penetrated deeply.

Collagen injections: A different technique altogether involves the injection of synthetic collagen to fill out lines and wrinkles, a procedure which is becoming increasingly popular in both the United States and Britain. In the past collagen from cow hide was used although now some products are entirely synthetic and tend to last longer before the need to repeat the treatment occurs. The presence of collagen can immediately improve the appearance of nose-to-mouth grooves, frown furrows, acne pits and depressed scars and it can also be used to plump-up narrow lips. Dilute forms can even be used around the eyes for crow's feet. Collagen injections can be quite an expensive option in the long term, however, because whichever form is used it is generally absorbed into the body within six months so that top-up procedures are required maybe two or three times each year.

Laser treatment: The very latest technique to treat fine lines and wrinkles involves carbon dioxide and the erbium: YAG lasers. Here the skin is painted evenly with the laser light, removing the lines and stimulating the replacement of older, damaged skin with a youthful, smoother surface. Lasers are very accurate, enabling deeper wrinkles and scars to be selected and treated separately.

Facelift: Finally, there is the surgical option, the facelift. Again, more and more women are enquiring about and opting for facelifts of which there are a number of alternative techniques being offered. A simple mini facelift is a basic operation where the surgeon cuts into the skin in a line beginning at the temples and running downwards in front of the ears and in behind them across the scalp. The skin is then lifted up off the facial structures, stretched taut and the extra skin trimmed off. Other procedures involve tightening up deeper layers of tissue beneath the skin to lift the eyebrows, take out bags around the eyes or enhance cheekbones. Such procedures require general anaesthetic, may cause possible complications and require a recovery period varying anywhere between two to twelve weeks. Facelifts are not procedures to be undergone lightly and thorough and competent counselling is an essential pre-requisite whenever any woman considers such an option.

Medical treatments for menopausal skin changes are summarised in the box below:

Colloidal oatmeal (Aveeno) and other emollients
Facial exercises
HRT
Cosmetic surgery:
– chemical peels
– dermabrasion
– collagen injections
– laser treatment
– facelifts

THINNING HAIR

Another possible consequence of declining levels of oestrogen at the menopause is a tendency for your scalp hair to become thinner. Your hair line can also recede slightly in much the same pattern as occurs in men at a younger age. Anything you can do to delay or prevent this hair loss is obviously very desirable. Medical help for hair changes which occur during the menopause are often of limited practical and cosmetic value. Someone whose expert opinion I value highly in this area is British Hairdresser of the Year, Charles Worthington. These are his top tips.

- Be aware that the texture of your hair may change. This awareness will help prevent further stress which in turn may have more adverse effects on the hair.

- Hair may become dull. Having a semi-permanent colour will add shine and vitality and give a healthier-looking frame to the face.
- Your hairtype may change from dry to greasy or greasy to dry. Changing your hair care products to suit your new hair type is essential.
- If hair is thinning, often a shorter cut makes it look healthier and thicker. Also, deeper, richer colours will give hair the appearance of being thicker – try to avoid blondes as they can make hair look thinner.
- Remember to invest in a good haircut as this will not only make your hair easier to manage, but is a great confidence booster.
- Scalp treatments are a good way of ensuring you have a healthy scalp, which in turn ensures you grow healthy hair.
- Pump up the volume in flat hair by using self-grip rollers. Place the rollers in dry hair, blast with a hairdrier and remove once they have cooled down.
- Using the correct brush to style your hair is both essential for the long-term health of your hair and for control. If you are unsure as to which brush to use, ask your stylist for advice.
- Comb conditioner through hair while it is wet and before you rinse. This way you will detangle the hair with the least amount of stress to the hairshaft, thus avoiding any unnecessary hair loss.

HEADACHES AND MIGRAINES

Due to the effect of oestrogen, migraines are more common in women than in men. Certainly fluctuations in hormone levels with normal menstrual cycles can trigger headaches of many different kinds in women. However, headaches tend to become much more common between the ages of 35 and 45 as women approach the menopause and overall levels of oestrogen begin to decline. Pre-menstrual headaches become particularly prominent during these years. It was once thought that the incidence of migraines declined after the menopause as oestrogen levels stabilised again, but research now shows that this is not necessarily the case. Some women have fewer migraines post-menopausally whereas others have more, and a small proportion of women actually find that their migraines begin at the menopause for the first time. In those women whose migraines have worsened, hormone replacement therapy may eradicate their symptoms or at least significantly reduce the frequency of attacks. Other factors other than hormones also play an important part. The anxiety and stress which may accompany the menopause can lead to tension headaches, and irritability and mood swings contribute too.

Treatment

There is no doubt that hormone replacement therapy can help many women whose headaches are more severe or more frequent before, during or after the menopause by ironing out fluctuating hormone levels. On the other hand hormone replacement therapy is also capable of producing headaches and migraines as a short-term side effect in vulnerable women. Because factors other than hormones may be responsible, many complementary therapies are worth considering. Acupuncture can enable the body to cope more effectively with depression, anxiety, irritability and stress. This treatment can alter the balance of the body's natural painkillers or endorphins, bringing about relaxation, comfort and peace. Aromatherapy also has a soothing effect, particularly when used simultaneously with massage. Lavender with camomile is wonderful for head, shoulder and neck massage as it eases tension and stimulates circulation. Clary sage is particularly good in helping to balance hormones. Osteopathy and chiropractic can ease out bunched muscles in the neck and shoulder regions, reducing the symptoms of tension headache and of nerve entrapment. It is particularly good in treating pinched occipital nerves in the neck which can transmit radiated pain over the top of the head to the brow and produce a sensation of intense sensitivity of the scalp itself. Spices, alcohol, smoking and caffeine are worth avoiding and a reduction in fat intake can be of benefit as all are potential trigger factors. Regular exercise and adequate sleep are both vital. Dietary supplements involving the B vitamin group and the antioxidants A, C and E are useful too. Because the causes of headaches and migraines are complex in and after the menopause, a homeopath would require a detailed consultation. Cimicifuga could be recommended for psychological symptoms whereas sanguinara might be suggested for headaches and hot flushes together. Homeopaths also use sage as apparently it has a good effect on sorting out hormone imbalances, whilst St John's Wort and Skull Cap are especially useful where anxiety and depression co-exist.

DECREASED MUSCLE TONE – JOINT AND MUSCLE PAINS

At the same time as menopausal women notice changes in the skin many notice that their breasts become smaller with a tendency to sag. The glandular tissue decreases in size as a result of oestrogen deficiency and the tone in the muscles of the chest wall, which support the breast tissue, is diminished with the result that the supportive tissue becomes slacker and looser. Muscles in the facial area, and the muscles of the pelvic floor and in the waist area begin to lose their tension and tone at the same time. This only serves to make the changing distribution of extra weight in the abdominal region even more noticeable. There are many reasons why muscles become weaker and less toned, the first one being simply a matter of age. As the years go by muscle bulk tends to be lost and the definition and hardness of muscles changes too. But certainly there seems to be a direct link between these changes and falling hormone levels. Studies using HRT in post-menopausal women have demonstrated a significant increase in muscle tone, confirming that falling oestrogen levels play a direct part. In addition, testosterone levels are falling at this time and since testosterone is a potent anabolic (muscle building) hormone, the combined effect of these endocrine changes is likely to result in alteration of muscle tone.

The cosmetic results are unwelcome enough but physical symptoms may manifest themselves in various ways. For many women aching and discomfort in the wrists, knees, ankles and back may be predominant features of the menopause. Back pain in particular, caused by laxity in the ligaments and joints of the vertebral column and loss of calcium in the bones, can lead to discomfort when sitting or standing for long periods of time. The stiffness in joints and a general feeling of weakness and malaise is common. Yet whilst these symptoms are often reported, no menopausal woman should assume that they are necessarily associated purely with the menopause. If there is a strong family history of osteoporosis with other risk factors being present, such as heavy smoking, low calcium diet and lack of weight-bearing exercise, consultation with the GP is a good idea so that a bone density measurement scan can be arranged if appropriate. Many forms of arthritis can manifest themselves in middle life too. Viral infections may sometimes produce quite severe joint discomfort, and both osteoarthritis, the wear and tear variety, and rheumatoid arthritis, the inflammatory variety, are not at all uncommon at a similar age. Tendons and ligaments around joints can easily be strained, and many minor injuries to joints take longer to settle and to repair themselves as time goes by. With decreased mobility the muscular-skeletal system is expected to become stiffer and less flexible too.

Treatments

It is a good idea to avoid sitting for more than an hour without taking a quick five-minute break. Standing for long periods of time too, particularly carrying shopping when wearing high heels, is asking for trouble. Plenty of stretching is beneficial, either as a simple bedroom routine or in a more structured form such as in a yoga class. Swimming is an excellent form of exercise as it uses all muscle groups and at the same time protects muscles, ligaments and joints from strain. Exercise generally is a must because it burns calories and turns them into energy using up stored fat cells in the body. Muscle activity creates warmth and lubrication to joints and releases chemical messengers within the brain known as endorphins. These are the body's natural opiates which promote a feeling of well-being and fulfilment in those who take physical exercise regularly. Maintaining physical activity in itself creates a continued sense of vitality and vigour. Ideally your routine should involve both aerobic activity to make the heart and lungs work harder, and also anaerobic activity involving strength-maintaining exercises using weights. Particular attention should be paid to bust and stomach exercises which maintain the female figure and help protect the back more than anything else. Another benefit of exercise is that it reverses the age-related shift in the lean body mass to fat ratio. As time goes by even if a woman's weight stays the same, the amount of fat in her body increases relative to the amount of muscle tissue or lean body mass. Exercise can reverse this, leading to a better toned body and a shaplier body which weighs the same. All women should realise that weight is not so much a problem as the overall amount of fat stored in the body.

Well-designed seating is important as slouching with a bent back in front of the television for hours on end will only lead to trouble. Well-designed stools of the Balans variety, where the weight is taken just below the flexed knees with the back in a vertical position, are available commercially and all office seating should be as ergonomically friendly as possible. Poor seating is one of the commonest causes of chronic back ache, with car seats being no exception. Relief of any joint or muscle discomfort using hot-water bottles or hot Epsom salt baths are useful, although the warmth supplied internally through exercising muscles is preferable. A comfortable mattress on the bed is vital, but bear in mind that orthopaedic beds are not strictly necessary as some can be extremely hard and will certainly not suit everybody.

For women worried about changes in their breasts, a well-shaped, well-fitting supportive bra, ideally fitted professionally free of charge at a major department store, can help a lot. Not only can cup size change but the chest measurement too can alter significantly after the menopause. Comfort and support are important.

In terms of diet, foodstuffs rich in calcium, vitamin D, oily fish and phytoestrogens are essential for helping to prevent osteoporosis and changes in muscle tone. Cod liver oil is a good supplement to take, along with natural herbal remedies such as black cohosh and meadowsweet which provide natural salicylates (the basic molecules of aspirin); Devil's claw, fennel, comfrey root and ginger may all prove helpful as well. Ginger in the form of capsaicin can be effective against rheumatoid arthritis by breaking down inflammatory proteins, easing pain, reducing swelling and stiffness and helping mobility. Even Carl Lewis, the Olympic gold-medal-winning sprint champion, now swears by it. Furthermore, glucosomine sulphate, an amino acid and derivative of glucose, is one of the essential building blocks in the production of both cartilage and connective tissue and though quite expensive it can significantly reduce pain and stiffness whilst promoting healing and restoring function. Chondroitin sulphate seems somewhat less effective but may also be worth a try.

Medical help
On the prescribed medicines front, hormone replacement therapy can confer considerable advantages in conserving muscle strength. A report for the Biochemical Society and the Medical Research Society in 1999 conducted a randomised trial of hormone replacement therapy to assess changes in muscle strength in post-menopausal women. They looked in detail at the adductor pollicis muscle, the muscle responsible for pulling the thumb towards the centre of the palm and then drawing it downwards so that it can touch the fingertips. Unlike the situation in men, where the age-related decline in muscle strength was gradual and started from the age of around 60, in the women in the trial who were not taking hormone replacement therapy there was a very sudden decline in muscle strength compared to

the women in the trial who *were* taking HRT. Similar results from other studies showed that thigh muscle strength was also preserved in women taking HRT after the menopause compared with women who did not. These results strongly suggest that oestrogen has an important role in maintaining muscle strength and that the use of HRT can partially reverse any weakness occurring at the menopause. Taking HRT for five to fifteen years after the menopause is likely therefore to result in increased muscular strength in addition to the increase in bone mineral density and protection against osteoporosis which HRT confers. Other options open to women with on-going muscle and joint discomfort include osteopathy and chiropractic. These therapies, once considered 'complementary' or 'alternative' remedies, have now been officially accepted into mainstream medical practice and can be extremely useful in easing the physical symptoms discussed above.

Surgery offers much more invasive and drastic choices, either in the form of cosmetic surgery to enhance breast shape and size, for example, or in the shape of orthopaedic surgery which can mobilise joints, remove slipped discs, ease inflamed tendons or even replace entire joints such as hips or knees.

CONSTIPATION

Constipation means different things to different people. Some women pass a motion every day as regularly as clockwork, other women can go for a week or longer throughout most of their lives before having to visit the loo. Either variation in bowel habit may be 'normal' for any one individual, however, and neither requires treatment in its own right unless symptoms occur. Constipation is medically defined as the infrequent passage of stools, usually three times a week or fewer, where there is pain or discomfort involved and where there may be incomplete evacuation of the bowels. Modern lifestyles, with a relatively poor intake of fibre-rich foods and a low level of physical activity, are obvious factors in the development of constipation with or without features of irritable bowel syndrome. Certainly women seem to suffer from constipation a great deal more than men and there may be factors other than female sex hormones involved. Women may be less physically active, and eat less fibre-rich foods. They may simply be busier and more distracted by dual careers and the attentions of children to be able to answer the call of nature every time.

Women also suffer twice as often as men from irritable bowel syndrome. This is where there is a combination of intermittent abdominal pain and irregular bowel habit, and where constipation alternates with diarrhoea in the absence of other diagnosed disease. Features include bloating, wind and a feeling of incomplete bowel emptying. There are other aspects of constipation and irritable bowel syndrome, especially in women, that deserve consideration. Clinical studies have shown that these symptoms may be associated with health problems unique to women, including breast lumps and pre-cancerous changes in breast tissue, and hormonal abnormalities. Falling oestrogen levels which occur around the menopause are particularly incriminated, but regularity of periods and operations for ovarian cysts or hysterectomies can also play a major part. Other factors include anal discomfort whilst making love, difficulty reaching orgasm, infertility and urinary incontinence. Women affected do not necessarily eat less fibre than other women but it seems increasingly likely that the bowel plays an important part in breaking down the female sex hormone oestrogen. Many women suffering from these conditions seem to have poorly co-ordinated and excessive contraction of the muscles around the lower end of the bowel, vagina and bladder.

Treatments

Troublesome constipation can lead to straining which in turn can make any problems with stress incontinence or haemorrhoids even worse. Since stress and tension may contribute to both constipation and irritable bowel syndrome any of the complementary therapies which deal with stress through relaxation techniques may be beneficial. Dr Peter Whorwell in Manchester has had considerable success treating irritable bowel syndrome with hypnosis, a safe and logical method of treating dysfunction in the digestive system caused by stress. Stress management courses are likely to pay considerable dividends, and acupuncture, aromatherapy and naturopathy are all complementary therapies well worth investigating.

Self-help
Self-help measures include establishing a regular routine of bowel habit, and increasing the intake of fibre in the form of wholemeal bread, cereals, fruit and vegetables. Increasing the intake of water to some four pints a day is imperative in helping the fruit and vegetables or the bran sprinkled on to other food to work. Slowly sipping a cup of boiled water first thing each morning can encourage a bowel movement, especially if it is followed by a cup of warmed prune juice. A breakfast to follow consisting of a dried-fruit compote containing figs, banana and dates is a particularly effective recipe. Another good suggestion is a banana blended in a liquidiser with a teaspoon of skimmed milk powder, a teaspoon of black strap molasses and a glass of milk. Regular exercise is another vital aspect of treatment as exercise is one of the most potent antagonists of the stress hormones adrenaline and nor-adrenaline known to man. During physical activity the digestive system slows right down and normal function all but ceases. Afterwards, however, it comes under the influence of the parasympathetic nervous system which reactivates the digestive processes and smoothly regulates its function. A weekly routine of 30 to 40 minutes exercise on three or four occasions is usually sufficient to bring about a significant change in symptoms. In addition, give up smoking and maintain a positive attitude at all times. Try to concentrate on feeling in control and then carry that through all aspects of your life whether in your career, at home or in relationships. As much as possible, avoid taking laxatives or antibiotics which in the long term can create more problems for the bowel.

Medical help

Medical investigations and treatment for constipation and irritable bowel syndrome involve the exclusion of significant physical disease. Constipation can sometimes be caused by an underactive thyroid gland, for example, a problem which is not at all uncommon at the age when most women approach the menopause. Other tests might include examination of a stool specimen, a barium x-ray or a sigmoidoscopy, a test which involves passing a narrow flexible telescope through the back passage into the bowel to examine the colon. These investigations are usually carried out when symptoms are moderate to severe and are important in ruling out conditions such as diverticulosis (where little pouches form in the wall of the bowel), ulcerative colitis and Crohn's Disease (which are inflammatory conditions of the lining of the bowel) and of course the very unlikely diagnosis of cancer of the colon. The latter is not commonly diagnosed at menopausal age but nevertheless occasional cases do arise and should be considered. If more serious conditions are ruled out and constipation or irritable bowel syndrome is confirmed, and when dietary manipulation and exercise prove inadequate in resolving symptoms, laxatives may be considered as a last resort to provide relief. Bulking agents consist of plant fibre such as bran, ispaghula and sterculia. There are also synthetic alternatives such as methyl cellulose. These increase the volume of the motions by absorbing water through the wall of the bowel and thereby softening the stool. These work slowly and gently. Such faecal softeners ease straining and are particularly useful in women with painful anal or rectal conditions such as fissure or haemorrhoids. Paraffin lubricates the passage of faeces but although it is safe and hardly absorbed it is not easy or pleasant to take and its use should be very temporary. Docusate sodium has a detergent action reducing surface tension and acts as a lubricant. There are also osmotic laxatives which draw fluid into the bowel and must be given with copious amounts of water. Lactulose and magnesium salts are good examples. Stimulant laxatives like senna are particularly potent but because they increase colonic motility they can cause considerable discomfort or even colicky abdominal pain. They work quickly but should be used with caution. For older women whose problems are located particularly within the rectum itself, glycerine suppositories are gentle and effective. Further help for patients can be obtained from the IBS Network or from the Digestive Disorders Foundation.

OTHER CHRONIC DISEASES

There are associations between the menopause and the occurrence of various chronic diseases and conditions. These include arthritis, disordered thought processes and Alzheimer's Disease, tooth loss and periodontal disease, cataract formation and even ovarian and colon cancer. These are not, however, common complaints at the time of the menopause, although as we shall see in Chapter 13, research into treating such disorders with hormone replacement therapy seems to be accumulating all the time.

NO SYMPTOMS AT ALL!

Reading about the catalogue of possible symptoms you might encounter during the menopause may be daunting. Remember, however, that it is highly unlikely that you would experience many of them and that most women, if they do notice any changes, are only aware of mild or moderate symptoms and even then only for a short while. Many women are delighted to experience no menopausal symptoms whatsoever. It might be helpful to refer at this point to the Menopause Assessment Scale in Chapter 6 to see how significant your own symptoms are in the great scale of things. Never forget that for each and every symptom of the menopause there is always an effective and relatively easy solution. So nobody in these enlightened times should have to put up with any physical inconveniences.

CHAPTER 4

PSYCHOLOGICAL SYMPTOMS AND
HOW TO TREAT THEM

That psychological problems are common around the time of the menopause is without question. What is less certain, however, is how many of these problems are related to the menopause itself and to decreased levels of circulating oestrogen and progesterone. I am personally very aware of relatively large numbers of women in my own surgery who complain of depression, anxiety and panic attacks, insomnia, mood swings, loss of concentration, confusion and libido changes in their mid-fifties; their loss of quality of life and suffering is almost tangible. Many of them attribute such symptoms to the menopause because it is what society has encouraged them to accept but men of this age also suffer similar symptoms despite the absence of a hormonal menopause.

There are many other factors which may be responsible for such symptoms at this time of life such as apprehension about impending retirement, marital difficulties and discord, responsibility for ill or dying parents and grown-up children leaving home. Particularly relevant to women are the understandable feelings of regret with the realisation that child-bearing opportunities are now for ever lost and that large sections of a society that surrounds them may regard them as being over the hill or socially redundant.

These negative and unhelpful cultural attitudes are very much part of the problem and they have undoubtedly coloured the way the medical profession regards the menopause. In fact the medical profession as a whole has been very guilty in the past of medicalising a normal life event. We should have moved on from the ridiculous notions of the Middle Ages where women's psychological state was inexplicably linked to their reproductive system and in particular to their womb. It is no coincidence that the prefix denoting the medical word for uterus and the irrational state of hysteria is exactly the same. Four hundred years ago the centre of all female psychology was invariably thought to be located in a woman's pelvis. Almost unbelievably doctors were still writing about the concept of 'involutional melancholia' as late as 1980. But sadness does not necessarily have to go hand in hand with the menopause.

Thankfully feminism and modern medicine have both moved on together towards a more rational and satisfactory understanding of common psychological symptoms in women.

Common psychological problems at the menopause

Depression
Anxiety
Insomnia
Mood swings
Memory loss
Poor concentration
Confusion

DEPRESSION

Depression is commonly reported at the time of the menopause. It can be a normal reaction to adverse circumstances, it can also be the main feature of a depressive illness with a sustained lowering of mood which may be disabling. There may be loss of interest or pleasure in the activities which a woman normally enjoys. She often feels that she cannot react emotionally to surroundings and events which are normally fulfilling. Sleep is often affected with the sufferer waking up two or three hours earlier than normal. The feeling of depression is often worse in the morning and the person concerned may feel physically slowed down and weary. Feelings of anxiety and agitation often accompany the depression. Some women also notice a significant loss of sex drive which may be the result of both psychological and physical changes.

Any menopausal woman experiencing any of these symptoms deserves a lengthy consultation with her doctor so that any underlying factors can be explored. An holistic approach, taking into account every aspect of mind, body and soul, is especially important in this situation. In a woman's late forties and early fifties many lifestyle changes are taking place. Grown-up children are fleeing the nest; rapid and unwelcome changes are being made at work in technology and working patterns; financial or marital difficulties may arise. There may also be very obvious physical discomforts arising from oestrogen deficiency such as troublesome hot flushes and night sweats, stress incontinence and menstrual irregularities. Is it any wonder that so many women of this age become unhappy and even clinically depressed? The fluctuations in oestrogen levels responsible for pre-menstrual syndrome and fluid retention are the same ones which can contribute to depression, although to what extent medical science is unsure. To make matters worse for many women, husbands and partners often have little insight into how a woman feels and may be even more clueless as to how to go about supporting her. As a result, many women report feeling that they are just existing rather than truly living. Interestingly, many medical studies lend support to a 'vulnerability theory'. In other words this means that women who have previously had depression may be at increased risk of mood disturbances during the menopause transition. Similarly, women who fear the events which the menopause may bring and who have low self-esteem and poor perception of the state of their physical health are more likely to report clinical depression at specialised menopause clinics. This may be one good reason why the medical profession attribute depression specifically to the menopause because the sample of menopausal women they see in the special clinics is unrepresentative of the population as a whole.

Treatment

Self-help
- A positive mental attitude and a constructive cultural outlook to the menopause is imperative in preventing and dealing with feelings of depression. Chapter 1 is devoted to such attitudes and highlights the importance of regarding the menopause as a change for the better.
- A problem shared is a problem halved. So talking to your partner and to friends is important in recruiting a level of understanding and support. Local and national self-help groups can both encourage and disseminate ideas about how to cope. Once a woman is diverted from a negative approach she can start to appreciate her new-found independence and wisdom, and not only dream her long-standing dreams and ambitions but turn them into reality.
- Dietary changes and supplements can be beneficial as can regular and varied types of exercise to break down stress chemicals and disperse feelings of irritability and aggression. Many doctors now prescribe exercise as a specific antidote to depression of all kinds.
- Hypericum (St John's Wort) has been proven in scientific trials to be of benefit in mild to moderate depression and, provided labelling instructions are carefully observed, is free at normal dosage of many of the worrying side effects of pharmaceutical medication.
- Herbal remedies worth experimenting with include black cohosh (cimicifuga racemosa) which can heighten energy and calm nerves. This is also useful for anxiety and stress. Sage (salvia officianalis) is also recommended for depression and mood changes as it is a natural tranquilliser rich in minerals such as magnesium and zinc. Sage helps to calm the nervous system and bring about peaceful sleep. Chastetree (vitex agnus castus) is also thought to be able to help eliminate depression and iron out fluctuations in mood. Dong quai (angelica sinensis) is another prized oriental plant treatment

helpful for depression, along with ginseng whose therapeutic action is particularly quick.

Medical help

Medically speaking, if depression is moderate to severe with pronounced tearfulness, early morning waking, persistent low mood and lack of energy, these self-help measures may not in themselves be sufficient. There is then a real risk in neglecting such deterioration with all the attendant consequences for both the woman and the members of her family. Professional counselling in the form of psychotherapy can be hugely beneficial and may be sufficient to resolve symptoms over a period of several weeks or months without the need for antidepressant medication. However, with persistent and severe symptoms modern anti-depressants which are well tolerated and quickly effective are the treatment of choice. Whether oestrogen and progestogen combi-nations have a significant effect on mood and well-being in post-menopausal women who are depressed is controversial. Some studies have shown significant improvements whereas others have not. Many doctors, however, believe that oestrogen therapy certainly improves a patient's response to antidepressants such as fluoxitene (Prozac), although hormone replacement therapy should not be relied on in itself to treat menopausal women with clinically significant signs of major depression. Advocates of natural progesterone might also bear in mind that as a natural antidepressant, treatment with this hormone in sup-pository form which, unlike progesterone creams, produces measurable changes in blood levels, is well worth considering.

ANXIETY

About 70 per cent of peri-menopausal women report significant symptoms of anxiety and about 30 per cent of these suffer moder-ately severe forms of it. Some research has suggested that anxiety is especially likely in women who have undergone hysterectomy.

All women appreciate that small amounts of anxiety can be biologically useful in that they increase efficiency, alertness and concentration. However, when the sense of apprehension and fear increases until it becomes out of proportion to a particular set of circumstances, it becomes a tremendous hinderance and can result in unpleasant physical symptoms such as nausea, palpitations and sweating. High levels of anxiety can also lead to the avoidance of circumstances which provoke it, leading to the onset of phobias such as agoraphobia. This can cause women to resist mixing with other people socially or even going shopping. Panic attacks may also be reported in menopausal women and are characterised by regular bouts of severe anxiety which are unpredictable and not confined to specific situations or circumstances. Panic arises when there is no objective danger, and in between such attacks the victim usually feels completely calm and free of apprehension. Headaches, chest pains, limb stiffness, breathlessness, irritable bowel syndrome, dry mouth, shaking and restlessness are all features of these types of symptoms.

Treatment

Many of the simple self-help coping strategies described above for depression apply to sufferers of anxiety too. Simple psychological support can often reveal underlying conflicts and difficulties for the patient, such as financial or relationship problems which may have contributed to the current situation. They need to be sorted out in themselves before the anxiety can really be brought under control. It is also important to discover whether the person concerned has been trying to escape from their anxiety and its symptoms through drinking too much alcohol, smoking more or even taking other recreational drugs. These will only have created additional problems rather than solving any of the underlying ones.

Stress relieving treatments using relaxation techniques can enable an anxious patient to recognise and relieve signs of muscular tension and to prevent irregularities in pulse rate or breathing which are otherwise involuntary. With this physical relaxation and ability to become calmer mentally, a more psychologically comfortable state often follows. Visualisation techniques will also help. For people with phobias, behavioural therapy is the mainstay of treatment. Graded exposure is an approach whereby the patient is progressively exposed to the feared situation one step at a time under specialist supervision. With a therapist's help patients learn to control their feelings of panic in a stressful situation and eventually they find they can cope with even the most alarming circumstances in apparent calm and control.

Peripheral to such psychological help, women should continue to exercise regularly, to find a reasonable balance of the energy they expend between their home life and their career, and they should take advantage of any help offered at Well Woman and Menopause Clinics if any exist locally. The best way to find these is to ask your own GP or their practice nurse. Nutritional therapy, meditation and yoga are all worth exploring too, as is massage and aromatherapy.

Tranquillisers are best avoided wherever possible as dependency on medicines such as diazepam (Valium), lorazepam (Ativan) and chlordiazipoxide (Librium) does potentially occur, particularly if they are used inappropriately and for extended lengths of time. The withdrawal symptoms associated with such dependency are every bit as bad, if not worse, than the original symptoms. Some of the antidepressants which have a mild sedating action can be useful in anxiety if depression is associated with it, though one of the most useful medicines for anxiety are the beta-blockers, such as propranolol, which ease physical symptoms like flushing, sweating and palpitations without affecting mental function or causing sedation at all. They are non-addictive but should be avoided in women with asthma, heart failure or diabetes.

INSOMNIA

Interrupted sleep is reported as commonly in menopausal women as hot flushes and night sweats. In fact these very physical symptoms may be partly responsible for any difficulty experienced in obtaining a refreshing night's sleep in the first place. In addition, aches and pains, stress incontinence and other physical symptoms of the change can all contribute. Hormonal factors and psychological ones play a part too, insomnia being often inextricably linked with depression or anxiety. Difficulty getting to sleep to begin with is often a sign of anxiety. The sufferer may feel extremely tired but her mind keeps mulling over the events of the day or worrying about future plans. Waking in the early hours of the morning can often signify clinical depression, the sufferer being able to get to sleep without too much trouble but then waking at four or five in the morning, tossing and turning for the rest of the night. The menopause itself often makes any underlying anxiety and depression worse in which case specific medical treatment for these conditions may be needed.

But a doctor should always be consulted before assumptions can be made that any sleepless nights are definitely due to the menopause itself and not to any other underlying condition. Scientific studies have shown that insomnia can in fact precede night sweats and other physical symptoms, and subtle brain-wave changes on an EEG (Electro Encaephologram) can be seen during sleep. This latter finding points to the fact that there is definite central nervous system involvement during the menopause in bringing about insomnia, and this may have something to do with the fact that oestrogen receptors have been located in brain tissue and that oestrogen deficiency may be partly responsible. Observation of sleep in menopausal women has also confirmed disturbance of the normal sleep cycle with a reduction in the amount of deep rapid eye movement (REM) sleep and attendant day-time fatigue the following day.

Treatment

Since insomnia is often aggravated by the physical symptoms of the menopause, treatment of these is important in alleviating sleep disturbances. Psychological factors such as anxiety and depression need to be corrected in their own right. Since hormonal, psychological and physical factors are all bound up in a complex pattern with sleeping problems, hormone replacement therapy could well be worth trying on an experimental basis. A high proportion of women find it significantly beneficial. There are, however, many simple self-help remedies which are worth adopting first. See box on pages 106–107.

Adopt the healthy sleeping tips in the box, together with other complementary therapies which may be beneficial. No matter what menopausal symptoms a woman suffers from, or how severe they may be, with a solid and fulfilling night's sleep she is much more likely to be able to confront those problems the next day, to adopt that positive mental attitude which is so essential to well-being.

MOOD SWINGS

Mood swings are commonly reported at the time of the menopause but to what extent they are governed by hormonal fluctuations rather than by the physical and psychological discomforts brought about by the menopause is in some scientific doubt. Traditionally, conventional doctors have always assumed that mood swings are an integral part of the hormone changes which can be measured during the change of life, although the women they have conducted their scientific studies upon in special menopause clinics have almost certainly been unrepresentative of the female population as a whole. It is a strong probability that if men (who are free of any measurable changes in hormone levels at the age of 50) were to suffer from hot flushes, insomnia, night sweats, incontinence and increasing weight, they too would suffer from irrational and unpredictable mood swings. All women are accustomed to accepting that there is a relationship between the hormonal events in their bodies and how they think and feel. They know that their female hormones are unique to them and are inextricably linked with body and soul. Alterations in a woman's hormonal balance, not just from day to day but from moment to moment, can alter the way she

Simple self-help remedies to aid sleep

1. Have a regular bed time at a reasonable hour. Keep the bedroom for sleep and love-making only. Routine always helps.

2. Avoid eating too late at night. Eating late leads to indigestion and heart burn. A full stomach also stimulates the intestine and produces extra body heat and sweating which clearly makes physical menopausal symptoms worse. Palpitations are also more likely.

3. Avoid excessive smoking and drinking in the evening. Both of these are strong stimulants which excite the nervous system, the very part of you which has to relax in order for you to get a good night's sleep. Although alcohol is actually a depressant, in pharmaceutical terms it will make you sleepy and tired to start with so you drop off to sleep but it has the distinct disadvantage of waking you up again half-way through the night when your body has overcome the alcohol's effects and when you need to empty your bladder.

4. Avoid other hidden stimulants. Caffeine in tea, coffee and cola drinks are likely to keep insomniacs awake, as may red wine, chocolate and cheese. Certain drugs and medicines act like nervous system stimulants too. Ask your doctor if anything you are currently prescribed could be keeping you awake, bearing in mind that appetite suppressants, asthma inhalers and pain killers are amongst the commonest. Even antidepressants can have this effect.

5. Take regular exercise daily. Exercise on a regular basis improves the quality of sleep, by influencing hormone secretions in the brain itself. Exercise tires you out physically as well as mentally but do remember to give yourself plenty of time to recover properly from its invigorating effects before settling down to sleep.

6. Make sure the bedroom is dark and quiet. A noisy room without blinds or curtains is certainly not conducive to staying asleep even if you get to sleep in the first place. Try to avoid extraneous noises such as traffic, loud music, babies crying and other people snoring. Fit dark curtains or blinds, keep doors

closed and if necessary, consider using ear plugs, which are available from most chemists.

7. Make sure the bedroom is warm but well ventilated. If your body is cold it sends survival messages to your brain, stopping you from sleeping, so adequate covers on the bed are obviously important. Avoid overheating however as this in turn can inhibit refreshing sleep and promote night sweats. Open the window for some fresh air.

8. Relax just before going to bed. Rid yourself of the day's worries by writing them down. Play a meditation tape such as my *Music for Wellbeing* tape on the Universal Classics label. Quiet reading, yoga and other relaxation techniques are also useful.

9. Invest in a comfortable bed. A comfortable bed to sleep on, especially if you have back problems, joint pains, neck stiffness or other physical symptoms, is vital in dropping off to sleep.

10. Spoil yourself. Have a warm bath before bed, preferably with lavender oil in it and perhaps some clary sage. Also prepare the bedroom by vaporising these oils or trying ylang ylang oil instead. Take a soothing bed-time drink such as camomile tea.

feels emotionally. It can colour her view of reality and impinge on whether she sees life as an exciting and stimulating challenge or a relentless source of stress leading to misery and despondency. This is why hormonal changes create such spiritual and emotional problems for women during pregnancy, for example, as part of pre-menstrual syndrome or during the menopause. If more women could see such changes in their moods as normal and as a natural reflection of the waxing and waning of endocrine influence on the female psyche perhaps less angst would be caused by these symptoms which may otherwise be generally regarded by society as undesirable.

It seems fair to assume that mild to moderate mood swings of a severity sufficient to cause reduction in the quality of life are definitely more likely to occur around the menopause. They are certainly much more likely to occur if depression is present or if the sufferer has had depression prior to the menopause or has approached the menopause with negative expectations of what it might have in store for her. Either way it is important that troublesome mood swings are treated. They can often make a woman who suffers from them feel angry with herself and guilty, and in severe cases this can affect relationships with other members of the family. Fortunately there is much that can be done to solve these problems.

Treatment

Self-help
Since stress is a major factor in bringing about mood swings, modifying the behaviour which makes a person more prone to stress is recommended. This involves learning about how to control emotions better and then practising drills which can enable a woman to change from being a stressed-out individual to becoming a calmer one. It takes time and practice but is well worth doing. You need to stop rushing about everywhere and concentrate on finishing one job at a time before moving on to the next. Try to wait patiently when you have to, without wasting energy by tapping your foot, wringing your hands, pulling your hair or biting your nails. Most women go through their middle life years 'poly-phasing', or in other words doing fifty jobs at a time. But prioritising those jobs and achieving the top two or three most important goals first can be helpful. It is also worth avoiding those situations which are particularly tiresome and irritating. Many women also set themselves un-necessary deadlines which generally serve to increase pressure further. Another good tip is to stop getting angry about things over which you have no control. You cannot change other people's behaviour however tiresome they may be, and attempt-ing to do so is just not worth the effort. So instead of boiling over in frustration because of having to suffer fools gladly, try to be a better listener. Remember that other people have problems from which you can learn; and remember also that, much as you might not want to acknowledge it, a highly stressed individual may sometimes hear what they least want to (but need to) from true friends or family. Try to become less competitive, and at all

times retain your sense of humour. Obviously it takes time and practice to change your behaviour in these ways so why not start by setting yourself some drills which are designed to encourage you to ease up.

Drills you can practise to help calm you down

Do everything more slowly.

Tell your partner and children you love them.

Do things which show your family you love them.

Observe the environment around you.

Consciously avoid physical manifestations of tension, such as gritting your teeth, tapping your foot or clenching your fist.

Listen to music rather than watching television.

Be prepared to question whether you are right or not.

Leave your watch off.

Take all your allowed breaks at work.

Practise listening to what other people have to say.

Ask a friend or colleague about their health and what is happening in their life.

Put thirty minutes in your diary for yourself every day.

Eat more slowly and have healthy lunches.

Practise being more assertive.

Try reading for thirty minutes every day.

Practise understanding and controlling your anger.

Spend less time talking about yourself in conversations.

Look up an old friend and enjoy old memories.

Take up a new interest.

Take a different route to work.

Soak in a relaxing bath for twenty minutes.

Enjoy a joke every day.

Write a letter or buy a small gift for someone.

Practise short relaxation routines.

Teach your children a new trick.

Book some time with your partner or give them a surprise.

These are just some of the exercises you can practise to start modifying the behaviour which makes you fraught with tension and more liable to mood swings. When you are aware of being ratty and irritable, practise some of the relaxation techniques described on pages 218–219 and try deep muscular relaxation or meditation instead.

Another major change you can make in order to iron out mood swings is to alter your diet. Try to ensure that a high proportion of your diet comes from fresh vegetables, raw seeds and nuts, fresh sprouted grains and seeds, as these can help to level out hormonal fluctuations, stabilise moods and improve the appearance of your skin, keep weight down and to some extent change your whole outlook on life. Concentrating on foodstuffs which are rich in phytoestrogens (see Chapter 11) can bring about a surprisingly dramatic improvement in how you look and feel within just a few weeks. Cutting down on fatty foods and foods with a high salt or sugar content is also likely to be beneficial for mood swings. Sugary snacks such as chocolate bars are well known to cause sudden changes in blood sugar and insulin levels leading to symptoms of irritability and moodiness.

In terms of medication, tranquillisers are best avoided except in very rare circumstances when mood swings are part of an acute anxiety state and when not using them would be more hazardous to health than using them. We know from the experiences of the 1970s and 1980s that hundreds of thousands of women were inappropriately prescribed tranquillisers and sedatives, leading to large numbers of women becoming dependent upon such drugs and suffering uncomfortable and distressing withdrawal symptoms when the drugs were discontinued. They should only ever be used in low dosage and in the very short term, say for up to two weeks, and even then preferably not taken every day. Antidepressants may have a place in treatment if the mood swings are part of a true and severe clinical depression but there are herbal alternatives to pharmaceutical drugs, including the use of hypericum (St John's Wort) which has been shown in clinical trials to be useful in mild to moderate depression. Other herbal treatments include camomile, valerian and evening primrose oil, while many women appear to benefit from Rescue Remedy and from stretching exercises such as yoga.

Medical help

As far as hormone replacement therapy is concerned, because of remaining doubts about whether mood swings are actually caused by oestrogen deficiency or not, the role of HRT in the treatment of mood swings during the menopause is still controversial. There is certainly *some* scientific evidence that improvement of mood occurs if HRT is taken but not all studies have come to such a conclusion. Overall, however, the consensus of opinion is that it does. Whilst it is possible that HRT improves mood swings by relieving definite symptoms of oestrogen deficiency, to what extent HRT is just a mental tonic which works by increasing a feeling of well-being by simply decreasing other menopausal symptoms still remains in doubt. It seems reasonable, however, that women who have other short-term symptoms of the menopause and who are particularly prone to severe and distressing mood swings should consider taking HRT so that any improvement in such psychological symptoms can be regarded as a substantial bonus.

Finally, since natural progesterone has a reputation for having calming and soothing effects on mood, it is recommended by its advocates as being just as useful during the menopause for mood swings as it is for women with pre-menstrual syndrome. Natural progesterone in suppository form or in those forms which can be obtained by mail order, such as oils, capsules, drops and skin creams, may therefore be worth trying by those women who do not wish to use traditional HRT.

MEMORY LOSS, POOR CONCENTRATION AND CONFUSION

In recent surveys 60 per cent of all menopausal women have reported feelings of not being able to concentrate and of confusion. A quarter of them suffer these symptoms in a mild to moderate form whereas 10 per cent apparently suffer severely. When you consider that we are talking about a quarter of the entire population, this is a problem of massive proportions. The kind of items that women find themselves commonly forgetting are essential items of shopping, messages they were given in the office and simple questions asked of them by their partners, such as where have they mislaid the car keys. None of these things is unique to the menopause and none of them is serious or life-threatening. But when small memory lapses cause an unnecessary irritation and frustration they in turn can lead to self-doubt and loss of confidence.

Some women actually attend their doctor's surgery and say that they feel as if they are going mad. At times they doubt their own sanity, so puzzled are they as to the degree of their un-predictable confusion. Their symptoms may be part of a wider picture, however, perhaps due to chronic fatigue as a result of insomnia or even poor nutrition and vitamin deficiency. These symptoms can also be due to the side effects of tranquillisers or antihistamines or even a result of physical discomforts attendant upon the menopause. Furthermore, chronic sleep disruption can result from something called obstructive sleep apnoea (OSA) and that can also adversely affect memory. In this condition, total relaxation of the soft tissues of the palate at the back of the roof of the mouth can obstruct the airways during sleep. Initially this causes snoring but eventually it can obstruct breathing altogether, resulting in increasingly greater efforts to breathe against the collapsed airway until typically the sufferer is awakened after about ten seconds of oxygen deprivation. Until the menopause men are eight times more likely to be affected by this than women although after the menopause the gender gap narrows considerably. This lack of breathing (apnoea) is especially common in women who are overweight since fatty tissue in the neck area puts extra pressure on the breathing passages. Those women who develop sleep apnoea tend to be excessively sleepy during the day, and after a while sufferers are unable to concentrate properly so their memory and judgement become impaired.

Depression and mood swings may often be a result of these factors. Clearly, if any of the above physical causes for the psychological symptoms of the menopause are present, they will need to be dealt with appropriately. Where no such causes are found hormonal influences may well be at play. The Victorians were wrong to believe that a woman's womb and her mental function are inextricably linked. But, interestingly, research conducted in 1996 discovered the presence of oestrogen receptors within the brain tissue itself as well as in the uterus, ovaries, bones and other organs of the body. This raised the question as to whether hormonal differences between men and women might explain why women out-perform men in tests of verbal fluency and when remembering details, but why men have a better sense of spatial orientation and can out-perform women on visio-spatial tasks of memory. This kind of speculation becomes even more interesting as it has been suggested that oestrogen may help post-menopausal women preserve their memory and even prevent the onset of dementia.

It has only recently come to light that oestrogen appears to be a powerful antioxidant, providing nerve cells in the brain with a chemical shield. Antioxidants mop up free radicals, the damaging particles resulting from environmental pollution, which can attack and destroy human tissues. Since 'oxidative stress' has been implicated in Alzheimer's Disease and Parkinson's Disease it is possible that oestrogen, both in natural and synthetic form, might successfully prevent and treat these neuro-degenerative disorders in the future. Several controlled clinical studies administering oestrogen to post-menopausal women have found that oestrogen does seem to enhance verbal memory and helps maintain the ability to learn new material. The oestrogen seems to increase the production in the brain of chemical neurotransmitters such as acetylcholine and dopamine. Some studies have also suggested that oestrogen has a protective effect on cognitive function and thinking power in women after the menopause. Also by its action on oestrogen receptors in the brain, deposits of a substance called beta-amyloid (the protein believed to be involved in the characteristic changes of Alzheimer's Disease) could be reduced.

Alzheimer's Disease is a degenerative brain disorder which manifests itself as a deterioration of memory and mental function, a state of mind often referred to as dementia. Its incidence increases with age, affecting more than 25 per cent of the over-eighties. The significant increase of Alzheimer's Disease last century is one reason why it is referred to as the disease of the twentieth century. Dementia, in fact, is one of the conditions associated with growing older that most of us fear most. No wonder so many people are following it with so much interest and hope the research into using HRT to combat Alzheimer's Disease will bear fruit.

Treatment

Supplements that may improve memory

1. Phosphatidylserine linked to the B vitamin group. This is a phospholipid which plays an important role in maintaining the integrity and fluidity of brain cell membranes. If there is a deficiency of folic acid or B12 or essential fatty acids, the brain may not be able to make enough phosphatidylserine. Low levels in the brain are associated with impaired mental function and depression. In a number of double blind studies which used phosphatidylserine in the treatment of age-related cognitive decline, Alzheimer's or depression, good results have been obtained in all of them. Statistical improvements were reported in mental function, mood and behaviour in the treated group as opposed to the group given the placebo.

2. Ginkgo influences at least two basic aspects of human physiology. It improves blood flow to the brain and to other tissues, and it also improves cellular metabolism. Scientific studies using 40 milligrams of a standardised ginkgo extract three times a day for a year showed significant improvements in short-term memory, alertness, mood disturbances, vertigo, headaches and tinnitus. Importantly there were no side effects reported and no interactions for commonly used heart and diabetes medication.

3. L-Acetylcarnitine. Carnitine is a vitamin-like substance responsible for the transport of long-chain fatty acids into the

---

energy producing units in human cells called mitochondria. L-Acetylcarnitine is a special form of carnitine manufactured naturally in the human brain which has been used in numerous scientific studies on the treatment of Alzheimer's Disease, senile depression and age-related memory defects. It acts also as a powerful antioxidant within growing cells and improves energy production within them. Together with phosphatidylserine, it has become popular with business people who want to stay sharp and on top of their work. It isn't therefore just for those with early stage Alzheimer's Disease or those believed to be getting early dementia, it is for people of all ages including women who have problems with memory and concentration at the time of the menopause.

4. Vitamin B Complex. Memory and concentration problems can also be the result of a chronically low intake of essential nutrients, amongst them B group vitamins. Thiamine is particularly crucial, as is B12.

In one of the most remarkable findings carried out to date, a sixteen-year study by researchers at the National Institute on Ageing at Johns Hopkins Bayview Medical Center showed that a history of oestrogen therapy in women after the menopause was associated with close to a 50 per cent reduction in the risk of developing Alzheimer's Disease. The same researchers also found that those women who were taking oestrogen showed fewer errors in short-term visual memory and of visual perception when compared to women who were not. Other studies have not, however, come up with quite such exciting results in favour of HRT, and in view of the fact that oestrogen therapy is capable of producing side effects, it is too early to state for sure that HRT should be prescribed preventatively for women with symptoms of confusion, memory loss or even a history of Alzheimer's. But it is another factor worth considering for women troubled by such symptoms who have other more definite reasons for being prescribed such therapy. In the meantime, there are many self-help measures a woman may adopt.

Self-help

- Anything that keeps the brain actively ticking over helps to keep somebody mentally alert and gets them into stimulating habits that will be neurologically rewarding for years to come. This is just as true for someone sitting at home all day as it is for someone in unchallenging employment.
- Joining an evening class or a local club, or even doing a university degree by correspondence course, can be beneficial; or if that seems a little self-indulgent what about putting your energies into something that will help others, such as volunteer work for your favourite charity or support group.
- Making new friends with people who care about the same things in life as you do is highly therapeutic.
- Another way of shaking off the inertia of middle age is to set some new goals. Plan that holiday of a lifetime, including visiting relatives abroad on their home territory. What about learning how to use the Internet and broadening your horizon that way?
- For specific memory skills remember to take notes. If you write it down you will not forget it. But write these notes down straight away because however good the idea may be, if you do not write it down immediately it will soon be forgotten.
- Get better organised too. If gathering and paying your bills is a task you find hard to remember, why not develop a specific place where you always keep your unpaid bills.
- Create a particular place where you always put your keys or your glasses or whatever the item is that you tend to lose most frequently.
- Make a conscious effort to exercise your memory every day, keep busy with crosswords and puzzles. If you are a morning person train your brain with word games and mind teasers before lunch, as morning people do their best work in the morning. If you are an evening person, you will probably retain learned material better as the day goes on, sometimes becoming very mentally astute towards midnight. But do not try to memorise everything you need to know all at once.

Make a habit of memorising a few things at a time and then having a break before memorising more.

- Use visual techniques as well. Imagine a mental picture into which you place the object you wish to memorise. If the picture remains always the same you will be surprised how many little extra objects you can hang within that mental picture without ever forgetting them. Memory tricks like this can work wonders for people whose memory is letting them down and, like all things in life, practice makes perfect.

NO SYMPTOMS AT ALL!

Many women are delighted to discover that they have escaped relatively scot-free from many of the psychological problems so often encountered by other women, and so often talked about in the press, which are associated with the menopause. Many women experience no problems whatsoever and I have only included a detailed look into potential symptoms in this chapter for completeness.

Most women will, however, notice a few inconvenient changes at the time of her menopause, whether of a physical or psychological nature, or possibly both. It would be worth referring to the Menopause Assessment Scale in Chapter 6 at this stage to see how mild or severe your own symptoms are in the great scale of things. The good news is that whatever your own experience of the menopause there is an effective and straightforward solution to any given symptom.

CHAPTER 5

SEX AND THE MENOPAUSE

Sexuality, Libido and Contraception

SEXUALITY

Sex and love-making is not the be all and end all in life and many loving couples still enjoy fulfilling and satisfying relationships with very infrequent sex or even without it. But for the vast majority of couples their sexuality remains an important aspect of the closeness between them and can be the key to how they transmit the affection they feel for the person they love. The ability to do this does not disappear either with age or as circumstances change. It is important that couples realise that their physical sex life is not over once the menopause is past, especially in view of the fact that these days women can expect to enjoy another third of their life beyond that period of time. It is quite possible to continue to enjoy happy and fulfilling sexual relationships and no woman should feel trapped because she is unable to consider sexuality positively or to explore the wide range of expressions of sexuality that are available. In fact, despite it being the case that sex drive naturally tends to reduce as we get older, physical contact need not diminish at all and should a woman choose to take HRT she could even find that her sex drive actually increases.

Negative attitudes surrounding the menopause and sexuality thereafter are widespread and very damaging. These beliefs can actually make it very difficult for women to get the help or advice they need because many health professionals and other advisors, along with many women themselves, share the mistaken belief that sex stops at the menopause if not some time before. Some women find it difficult to accept that people in later life have sexual desires and drives. Some even find it inappropriate or even distasteful. Many women are encouraged to take up new interests which may be intellectually stimulating or of value to the community and which keep idle hands and minds employed. Yet bizarrely there still remains a taboo on translating that into the development of personal relationships and into the area of sexual exploration. In fact until very recently sex and sexuality for many women was entirely associated with fertility and their child-bearing years. If a woman's sex life had previously been unsatisfactory the arrival of the menopause was a time when with great relief she could say 'thank goodness that's all over', and discontinue any sexual activity completely.

A woman's enjoyment of sex in her younger years, before the menopause, will certainly have a strong bearing on her attitudes towards sex afterwards but for those women who have always enjoyed the closeness and intimacy that love-making brings, both emotionally and physically, there is absolutely no reason whatsoever why the menopause should deprive them of it. There is no single physical or psychological symptom associated with the change that cannot be overcome, and those women who feel that sexual intimacy is an essential part of their lives should strive hard to preserve it for many years to follow.

Touching and Intimacy

After the menopause and the last flushes of youth, touching and intimacy become more important than the physical pleasure of intercourse. This need to touch and be touched both physically and emotionally is well worth nurturing. This contact offers reassurance and comfort, and the opportunity to show tenderness, companionship and love. Intimacy involves giving and receiving love, and exposing some small part of ourselves to another person we trust more than anybody else. This vulnerability and trust is pivotal in any loving relationship. As the years go by the focus on genital stimulation in a sexual relationship (which is more important in the very young) tends to become overtaken by the emotional, physical, social and spiritual ingredients of love as relationships become more mature. There are many expressions of love other than sexual intercourse, and all can boost confidence and enhance feelings of self-esteem and worth.

Reduced Sexual Function

Sexual activity tends to diminish with advancing years, or should I say (somewhat less pessimistically) with diminishing youth. Large surveys conducted amongst European countries and in the United States of America show that 70 per cent of women aged 45 to 54 are sexually active, falling to 60 per cent among those aged 55 to 64. Whether part of the age-related reduction in sexual behaviour is due to the menopause in itself is uncertain, but there is reason to believe that certain menopause-related symptoms definitely interfere with sexuality. These would include all the physical and psychological symptoms that may be encountered.

Troublesome Symptoms of the Menopause

There are undoubtedly a number of symptoms related to the menopause, of both a physical and a psychological nature, which can temporarily hamper a woman's ability to enjoy a fulfilling sex life. Night sweats and hot flushes, for example, can be completely counterproductive to relaxation and romance. Night sweats produce an intolerable feeling of heat, sometimes accompanied by profuse sweating, even a feeling of claustrophobia. If the victim has to throw off the bedsheets and throw open the windows at the best of times, having her partner lying on top of her is hardly going to improve matters.

Another definite symptom of the menopause caused by relative oestrogen deficiency is vaginal dryness and thinning of the vaginal lining. See Chapter 3. This lack of lubrication and support for the vaginal walls can lead to a reduction in arousal during sex, and increased friction in turn may promote soreness, burning or irritation. Irregular periods can make the timing of spontaneous love-making awkward and sometimes embarrassing, as can stress incontinence which can occasionally arise during love-making itself. Women who have undergone hysterectomy but who were not fully counselled prior to their operations may retain negative attitudes about their sexuality and femininity as may women who have had a mastectomy. These psychological trains of thought can have a very potent effect on diminishing a woman's ability to enjoy sex. Other women lack confidence about their on-going attractiveness for their partner as a result of weight gain or redistribution of weight away from their breasts and towards their waistline. Some are conscious of changes in the shape of their breasts and of drier skin, although the fact that their partner's physical appearance is also likely to have changed may seem almost irrelevant.

Compound these physical symptoms with psychological ones such as mood swings, insomnia and depression, and it is little wonder that sexual function seems to diminish at the menopause and thereafter. Yet many women seem to overcome these difficulties quite easily and carry on enjoying a satisfactory love life for many post-menopausal years. Many physical problems can be alleviated so they shouldn't necessarily have to cause a hindrance to sex, and some women even report an enhanced love life. Now that teenage children have grown up and left home there is more freedom and independence to become more intimate with one's partner again, and release from any fears of pregnancy and from periods can actually lead to a renewed and revitalised love life.

Making the Most of It

It is now clear that women have at least the same ability as men to enjoy sex, plus the additional advantage of retaining their capacity to have several orgasms, one after another, until much later in life. Men, when they are young, are capable of making love several times a night but as they get older they are satisfied with love-making only once or twice a week, or even much less.

Many women discover a renewed or even redoubled libido when they are started on hormone replacement therapy and not uncommonly report that their husbands can no longer keep up with their sexual demands! For many post-menopausal women, the fact that their husbands take longer to reach a climax becomes a bonus. For the woman it makes love-making far more enjoyable than when they were younger and everything seemed to be all over in a matter of breathless seconds. Although this can make men anxious, more prolonged love-making can be turned to advantage by providing time for both partners to explore new sensations and enjoy a variety of feelings. (In terms of any physical and psychological symptoms, all of them can be improved using specific treatments which are discussed in Chapters 3 and 4. A positive attitude also helps to dis-inhibit women who have been brainwashed into thinking that life, including sex life, stops after they hit the menopause.)

LIBIDO

Many women complain that after the menopause they simply lose their desire for sex. Those women who used to initiate sex with their partners may determinedly avoid it, although many report that once they do make love they are surprised to find that they actually do still enjoy it. If a woman's partner maintains his normal interest in her but is constantly rebuffed in his advances this can lead to an understandable feeling of rejection and in turn may bring about relationship difficulties. Reduced libido in peri-menopausal women remains a tough therapeutic egg to crack and one which millions of women throughout the world and, for commercial reasons, the pharmaceutical industry would dearly love to find a solution to. Since time immemorial, the search for aphrodisiacs capable of stimulating erotic desire and enhancing sexual performance has been intense. Various substances used as love potions over the centuries include honey, ginseng, ginger, strychnine, rhinoceros horn and oysters. Alcohol has been used to encourage sexual desire by removing inhibitions, and marijuana, yohimbine (a chemical obtained from the bark of the West African yohimbine tree) and amyl nitrite have all been used for the purposes of stimulating desire. Unfortunately none of them have been shown to have any measurable effect and some, such as alcohol, may actually impair sexual performance.

The good news, however, is that more recent work using natural herbs does seem to suggest that female sex drive can be boosted. Whether the menopause, childbirth, stress or merely the presence of children is the cause of diminished libido, a mixture of standardised extract of Muira Puama combined with Ginkgo Biloba has shown considerable success in early studies. According to recent interim results, 67.5 per cent of women tested experienced a net improvement in the quality of their sex lives using this combination, including a greater frequency of erotic thoughts and desire for sex, as well as a better ability to achieve orgasm, and more intense orgasms, in twice as many cases. For women not keen on hormone replacement therapy, experimentation with such herbal remedies may be attractive. Other experimental work on sildenafil, otherwise known as Viagra, the revolutionary medication for male impotence, also suggests that libido in women may be enhanced by using it. It is possible that the increase in blood flow to the genital area in women may lead to increased arousal during intercourse and better lubrication, but further studies are awaited at the present time.

Hormone Therapy

There is no controversy whatsoever about the benefits of hormonal treatment for sexual discomfort in a post-menopausal woman with vaginal atrophy. Vaginal dryness, lubrication, soreness, irritation and a vulnerability to bacterial infection or thrush may all be vastly improved by using hormone replacement therapy with oestrogen. Other physical symptoms which may also predispose to lack of enjoyment of sex, such as hot flushes, may also respond to such HRT. But whether diminished sexual desire, arousal, orgasm or overall sexual satisfaction would directly benefit from oestrogen treatment is not definitely known. Advocates of HRT can be loud and vociferous about the perceived benefits. Media coverage in magazines and newspapers often cites well-known personalities boasting of their renewed sexual aggression and enjoyment when HRT is taken. Yet there is no sound evidence that HRT alone brings this about. I know of at least one famous female celebrity who boasts that she has sexually devoured at least four toyboys on the strength of HRT. Unfortunately, however, this level of expectation of HRT is likely to lead to massive disappointment!

It is likely that testosterone has a more significant effect on decreased libido than oestrogen. Results showing that testosterone improves sexual desire come from studies on women who have had their ovaries removed for one reason or another and then received high doses of testosterone. In these women their levels of testosterone falls by 50 per cent soon after their surgery. In women having a natural menopause, however, testosterone levels fall by much smaller amounts, and to what extent testosterone treatment will help them with loss of libido is uncertain. Several studies have shown that low dose testosterone is effective and very well worth trying for postmenopausal women reporting low sexual drive. Whilst GPs are generally unfamiliar with such therapy, specialists might well consider using a short duration trial of 5mg of oral methyl testosterone together with conjugated equine oestrogens for this purpose. But if testosterone is used it is best used under supervision in low dose and in short duration to minimise any risk of side effects. These may include hair loss on the head, acne, unwanted body hair, weight gain, headaches, nausea and raised levels of blood fats. The same side effects apply to the alternative to oral testosterone therapy, namely testosterone implants, which can be inserted every six months and which have proved of particular value to women having a surgical menopause through removal of both ovaries.

CONTRACEPTION

As you approach your menopause, the diminishing supply of responsive egg follicles within your ovaries means that you become less fertile. See Figure 10. Well over a third of women aged 45 to 50 have menstrual cycles which miss ovulation completely. Because ovulation is irregular, periods too become irregular, and this is a normal occurrence for about four years prior to the menopause itself. Only about 10 per cent of women stop periods suddenly, the remainder experience erratic menstruation for some considerable time. Oestrogen levels are also unpredictable. Whilst they drop by up to 80 per cent in the year or so after the menopause, hormone fluctuations continue for some time and the last few ovarian follicles may still respond. Because of this there remains a small and unpredictable chance of conception and pregnancy even at and slightly beyond the menopause. Whilst many women will have changed to more appropriate methods of contraception in their forties, which reflect diminished fertility and the decreased need for safety, other women mistakenly assume that their child-bearing days are already over and omit contraception altogether. At the age of 45, Cherie Blair, the Prime Minister's wife, was certainly not alone in perhaps assuming her fertility at 45 to be negligible, only to be delightfully surprised to find that she was pregnant. Late pregnancy can and does happen and for this reason it is important, even beyond the menopause, to be correctly advised about contraception. The recommended advice is as follows: Women over the age of 50 should use contraception for 12 months after their last period. Women who are under 50 when they have their menopause should continue to use contraception for two years. Finally, if a woman has started taking hormone replacement therapy before her last period, she should continue using contraception until the age of 53 to be on the safe side. This is because HRT is different in hormonal content to the oral contraceptive pill and does not have a contraceptive action of its own.

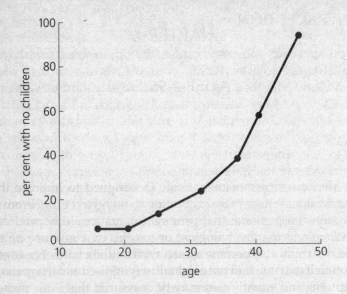

Figure 10 **The chance of older women not having a baby**

IN SUMMARY

There is now no earthly reason why women cannot continue to enjoy a happy and satisfying sex life during and after the menopause if they want one. Every psychological and physical inconvenience encountered and which may get in the way temporarily can be overcome so that couples can remain close, intimate and loving in every possible sense.

Take a look at the Menopause Assessment Scale in the next chapter to see just how significant are any symptoms which you have and which relate to sex and sexuality. The good news is that for every possible problem there is always a satisfactory and effective solution.

CHAPTER 6

YOUR MENOPAUSE ASSESSMENT SCALE

The Menopause Assessment Scale is designed to indicate the severity of symptoms you encounter at any given time. From it you may see at a glance that your symptoms are either predominantly physical, psychological or sexual, or a mixture of all three. You may also become aware, whilst filling it in, of changes in yourself that you had not originally recognised as menopausal symptoms and equally you may be reassured that your menopause is not as bad as you had once imagined it was. The assessment is only a rough guide, of course, as many other disorders can contribute to several of the listed symptoms, but for a woman in good general health and on no medication it can certainly act as a guide for discussion with her doctor, and it can indicate what kind of treatment might be most suitable and appropriate for her. Stephanie has filled in her assessment and we can use it as an example.

For each of the possible symptoms she might encounter during her menopause she scores zero if symptoms are absent, 1 for mild symptoms, 2 for moderate symptoms, and 3 for severe symptoms. In other words she gives each listed symptom a score ranging from 0 to 3 but she attaches only one score to each horizontal column. Read about her own experiences of the menopause and look at how she has completed her assessment, and then complete your own assessment in a similar way using the scale on page 130. Once you have totted up your total score refer to the recommended treatment guide on page 131.

STEPHANIE'S MENOPAUSE ASSESSMENT SCALE

	NONE (0)	MILD (1)	MODERATE (2)	SEVERE (3)
PHYSICAL SYMPTOMS				
Hot Flushes				3
Night Sweats				3
Palpitations		1		
Irregular Periods			2	
Cystitis/Stress Incontinence	0			
Vaginal Dryness			2	
Vaginal Irritation			2	
Weight Gain			2	
Thinner Skin & Hair		1		
Headaches	0			
Loss of Muscle Tone		1		
Fatigue/Joint Pains		1		
Constipation/IBS	· 0			
Periodontal Disease	0			
PSYCHOLOGICAL SYMPTOMS				
Insomnia			2	
Depression		1		
Anxiety		1		
Poor Memory/ Concentration	0			
Decreased Libido			2	
Mood Swings		1		
TOTAL SCORE	0	7	12	6 = 25

Stephanie is 51 and has been experiencing severe hot flushes and night sweats for several months. The hot flushes bother her about three or four times a day, lasting between two and three minutes, bringing her out in a florid rash on her face and neck, and making her damp with perspiration. At night she often has to throw the duvet off the bed and fling open the window for air. Occasionally she gets palpitations when she feels her heart flutter as the hot flushes come on. Her periods have been unpredictable for a couple of years and she has noticed a definite lack of vaginal lubrication with consequent itching and irritation down below. She says these factors have certainly contributed to her loss of sex drive. She just does not feel like initiating lovemaking with her partner at the current time. 'If he doesn't like it,' she says, 'it is just tough!'

Her weight has increased by ten pounds in the last 18 months, she hates those tell-tale wrinkles, and she tries to avoid looking in the mirror at her once lovely breasts which, she feels, are beginning to sag. If only she did not feel so tired and have so much to do life would be easier – a problem only made worse by her recent inability to get a good night's sleep.

Stephanie admits she feels somewhat 'down' about all these changes, and not a little anxious about what the future holds in store for her. For his part her partner, Tom, is devoted to Stephanie and has told her in no uncertain terms that he loves her and will always do all he can, despite her unpredictable and rather alarming mood swings, to tide her through this challenging time.

Stephanie has filled in her assessment based on her above symptoms and it gives her a score of 25 which puts her squarely in the category of a severe menopause based on the treatment guide on page 131. Thankfully, not many women will experience as many difficulties as Stephanie has during her menopause but most will benefit from advice, support, lifestyle changes, dietary adjustment, complementary therapy and possibly hormone replacement treatment.

Carry out the self-assessment yourself to see exactly where you stand.

YOUR OWN MENOPAUSE ASSESSMENT SCALE

	NONE (0)	MILD (1)	MODERATE (2)	SEVERE (3)
PHYSICAL SYMPTOMS				
Hot Flushes				
Night Sweats				
Palpitations				
Irregular Periods				
Cystitis/Stress Incontinence				
Vaginal Dryness				
Vaginal Irritation				
Weight Gain				
Thinner Skin & Hair				
Headaches				
Loss of Muscle Tone				
Fatigue/Joint Pains				
Constipation/IBS				
Periodontal Disease				

	NONE (0)	MILD (1)	MODERATE (2)	SEVERE (3)
PSYCHOLOGICAL SYMPTOMS				
Insomnia				
Depression				
Anxiety				
Poor Memory/ Concentration				
Decreased Libido				
Mood Swings				

TOTAL SCORE

Now tot up your total score and, depending on which category you fall into, find out what your next course of action should be.

What Your Assessment Score Means in Terms of Treatment

Score 0–6
This is a pre-menopausal score as six mild symptoms could easily be experienced in an otherwise healthy woman at any time.

Talk over your symptoms with your GP especially if they are persistent or if they become worse and he or she may well be able to prescribe an appropriate treatment.

Pay attention to a healthy diet and lifestyle, and take advantage of well-woman screening.

Score 7–13
You are experiencing enough symptoms now for the menopause to be noticeably affecting your quality of life. You do not have to grin and bear it any longer.

Go for well-woman screening, talk to your doctor about your problems and consider blood tests to measure hormone levels (see Chapter 10). Discuss the value of HRT in the prevention of osteoporosis and heart disease.

A diet rich in phytoestrogens is recommended along with self-help measures and complementary therapies to help with these mild symptoms.

Score 14–20
You are in the midst of a moderately severe menopause which will be taking its toll on your enjoyment of life and your ability to cope with normal daily events.

Go for well-woman screening and talk to your doctor about all aspects of your life and how you really feel. Blood tests and other investigations may be appropriate. Discuss the pros and cons of HRT and your own feelings about it.

A diet rich in phytoestrogens is recommended along with

self-help measures and complementary therapies to help with these symptoms. Consider HRT for complete control of symptoms and long-term protection.

Score 21 and above
Unfortunately you are one of the unlucky ones destined to go through an uncomfortable and turbulent menopause unless you have treatment for it. Even with the most positive mental attitude you are likely to feel below par without help of some kind.

Go for well-woman screening. Make an appointment with your doctor and be frank and open about how you feel. Talk to a local self-help group, the Amarant Trust or Women's Health Concern (see Useful Addresses). Have any necessary tests and find out all you can about HRT and its alternatives.

A diet rich in phytoestrogens is recommended along with self-help measures and complementary therapies to help with these symptoms. Consider HRT for complete control of symptoms and long-term protection.

PART TWO

CHAPTER 7

HEART DISEASE AND THE MENOPAUSE

Until recently the vast majority of women believed that the consequences of the menopause were relatively short-lived and more of a nuisance than anything else. Many doctors and nurses shared this opinion. But in recent years there has been a growing realisation that the long-term consequences of the menopause are even more important than the events which occur within a year or two of stopping periods, and that understanding, preventing and treating problems such as heart disease, breast cancer and osteoporosis is now an essential part of modern medical care. Thankfully, just as it is possible to alleviate satisfactorily all short-term menopausal problems, we are now able to prevent and treat these more serious and long-term problems as well. Let's start with heart disease.

Coronary heart disease is the biggest single killer of postmenopausal women, and more women in Britain will die from heart disease than from any other medical condition. The coronary arteries are the major blood vessels which feed the heart and supply it with nutrients and oxygen. Partial blockage of these arteries leads to chest pain known as angina, a sensation of pressure behind the breast bone typically associated with strenuous activity, which can radiate into the arms, upwards into the throat and tongue, or towards the back. Total sudden blockage in the coronary arteries deprives part of the heart muscle of all oxygen, leading to the death of a portion of the heart muscle or in other words a heart attack. As well as pain and breathlessness, nausea, heart failure and abnormal heart rhythms can develop as a result of these two forms of coronary artery disease. Regrettably, nearly 20 per cent of older women who suffer heart attacks or cardiac arrest will die suddenly as a result.

Amazingly, the first ever medical report describing a heart attack was written in 1912 yet heart disease has now become epidemic amongst Western societies where decreased exercise and a diet rich in saturated fat is taken. Whether women survive heart disease depends on how severe the condition has become, whether they smoke, whether they have diabetes, whether their blood pressure is raised and whether their blood cholesterol levels are high. Much depends on the type of treatment they take as well. Sudden death is one result of coronary heart disease, but it can also lead to a wide range of disabilities and limitations in a woman's daily activities. For a start she will be unable to perform strenuous activities. In its most severe form heart disease will cause patients to become essentially bed-ridden and unable to engage in any social or physical activity because of disabling chest pain or problems with breathing. As time goes on sufferers can experience either a gradual decline or a stepwise deterioration punctuated by critical events such as further heart attacks or strokes.

Who is at Risk of Heart Disease?

For both men and women there are a number of factors which increase the risks of developing heart disease in the future. These include:

Risk factors for heart disease

increasing age
having a family history of heart disease
being diabetic
being a smoker
being overweight
having high blood pressure
coming from a lower socio-economic class
having elevated cholesterol levels
taking little exercise

Men generally develop coronary heart disease some ten years before women do and tend to die of it some 20 years earlier. This is because women are relatively protected until the menopause by their female sex hormones. Without such protection women would be more likely to have coronary heart disease. There are additional risk factors for some women.

Additional risk factors in women

premature ovarian failure
having both ovaries surgically removed before the natural
   menopause
lack of hormones due to genetic conditions such as Turner's
   Syndrome or other conditions caused by chromosomal
   aberrations

Looking at all the above risk factors, it is obvious that some are impossible to change. You cannot, for example, change your genetic make-up, you cannot change who your parents were. You cannot defy nature and cease to become older, nor can you have any direct influence over failure of ovarian function, either at the menopause or before it due to unavoidable surgery. You can, however, make other important changes to minimise your risk:

- You can make sure that your blood pressure is measured on a regular basis and kept within normal limits.
- You can stop smoking or cut down.
- You can keep your weight within normal limits for your height.
- You can take more exercise and you can take greater efforts to keep blood sugar levels within the normal range if you are diabetic.
- You can also have your cholesterol levels checked and adjust your lifestyle so that the ratio of your good and bad cholesterol levels remain healthy.

Cholesterol

Cholesterol is an essential component of the body and is used by cells for all kinds of functions, including the manufacture of hormones and the maintenance of cell membranes. Twenty per cent of the cholesterol in the body comes from the food which we eat and the rest is made naturally by the body itself, mainly in the liver. In the bloodstream cholesterol is transported by lipoproteins which are combined fat and protein molecules and which are of either high density or low density. High density lipoproteins (HDLs) are known as 'good' cholesterol because these lipoproteins attach to cholesterol in the walls of arteries and ferry it away back to the liver again for excretion. Low density lipoproteins (LDLs) are considered 'bad' because they transport cholesterol in the opposite direction, allowing cholesterol to build up in the walls of the arteries as fatty deposits, one of the major determinants of future heart disease. Elevated levels of HDL cholesterol are therefore seen as desirable because they are associated with less heart disease. High levels of LDL cholesterol, on the other hand, are considered undesirable for the opposite reason. The healthiest and most ideal ratio for a person to have when their blood is measured is three parts HDL to one part LDL, and there are many things that you can do to improve this ratio and reduce your overall level of circulating cholesterol.

- You can avoid fried foods and limit your intake of fatty meats and other foods which are high in saturated fat. Oily fish such as mackerel, tuna, herring and salmon are healthier alternatives.
- You can also eat plenty of fresh fruit and vegetables which are rich in calcium, magnesium and potassium.
- By reducing the amount of salt in cooking or added to food as a condiment, high blood pressure can also be avoided.
- Taking more aerobic type exercise can also help to burn up excess levels of cholesterol as energy.
- Avoiding smoking is a vital factor as smoking contributes in a major way to heart disease.

- Avoiding stress as much as possible will also help.
- Taking extra antioxidant supplements like vitamins A, C and E and minerals such as selenium are recommended.
- Another important way of avoiding the risk of heart disease after the menopause is to consider hormone replacement therapy.

HRT

It is known that, because of the presence of female sex hormones prior to the menopause, women are relatively protected against coronary heart disease until later in life. The evidence for this comes mainly from the fact that women who have had their ovaries surgically removed early have double the risk of coronary heart disease unless they take HRT, which significantly reduces it again. Confirmation comes from the fact that in women who take HRT after the menopause the chances of developing coronary heart disease are drastically cut by up to 50 per cent. How does HRT achieve this? The protective effect of HRT seems to begin shortly after therapy is started and persists for several years even after a woman stops taking it. One of the ways in which it is thought to work is by improving blood cholesterol levels. HRT reduces bad cholesterol (LDL) and increases good cholesterol (HDL). So great is this effect that recent guidelines for doctors on controlling cholesterol levels state that HRT should be seriously considered for post-menopausal women because the reduction in levels of LDL and the increase in levels of HDL are 15 per cent equally. In addition, HRT has a favourable effect directly on the blood vessels which supply the heart. Oestrogen increases the production of a substance which relaxes the blood vessel walls and helps to keep the coronary arteries wide open. These hormones can also decrease production of a substance called 'plasminogen activator inhibitor', which is associated with hardening of the arteries (atherosclerosis) and heart attacks.

Whereas the evidence to support the beneficial effect of HRT is strong, some authorities question the validity of these findings. Some doctors believe that in the studies carried out there has been 'selection bias', a phenomenon resulting from the fact that if only healthy women are given HRT in order to assess its efficacy in trials then the apparent health benefits will simply reflect this initially biased selection of healthy women. In fact, when all factors were taken into account by epidemiologists, and detailed checks had been made for any differences between women who use and women who do not use HRT, there remained a substantial protective effect of between 30 per cent and 40 per cent, which still remains particularly impressive. So much so that doctors throughout Europe who specialise in treating the menopause now believe that its beneficial effect on the cardiovascular system means that women with raised cholesterol levels or high blood pressure, along with women smokers and diabetics, should all be offered HRT as a preventative treatment, particularly if there is nothing in their family history to suggest that they are at greater risk of breast cancer. Since more women will die from heart disease than from any other condition post-menopausally, and since the risk of breast cancer is relatively small as a result of taking HRT, this would certainly be the consensus of medical opinion at the current time.

CHAPTER 8

OSTEOPOROSIS AND THE MENOPAUSE

Osteoporosis is a condition in which the bones have lost much of the supporting structure which keeps them strong. It is a progressive generalised disorder of the skeleton characterised by low bone density and deterioration in the micro-architecture of bone tissue, resulting in greater bone fragility and susceptibility to fractures. Osteoporosis is sometimes called brittle bone disease because certain parts of the skeleton become extremely vulnerable to fractures either from minor trauma or sometimes from no trauma at all. It is still a common sight to view elderly women struggling down the street uncomfortably hunched over their shopping, revealing their obvious dowager's hump. The more fragile bones in their spine have become wedged at the front so that their back becomes bent forward, and they have lost several inches in height as a result of gradual spinal compression. Minor tumbles, even in relatively young women, often result in broken wrists, hips and spines, and sometimes merely coughing, sneezing or laughing can crack a severely osteoporotic rib or other bone. (Figure 11 shows strong dense bone and fragile osteoporotic bone.)

Bone is living tissue and is constantly changing. Old worn-out bone is broken down by cells called osteoclasts and replaced by cells known as osteoblasts which construct new bone. This whole process of renewal is called bone turnover. In childhood, osteoblasts work most efficiently, allowing the skeleton to increase in density and strength. At this time bone grows rapidly and the entire skeleton can renew itself within two years. By adulthood bone turnover becomes slower and it takes seven to ten years to renew the entire skeleton. By the age of about 18 the longbones of the body stop growing so quickly in length but

Normal bone cross-section

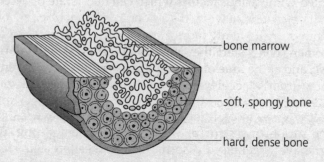

— bone marrow

— soft, spongy bone

— hard, dense bone

Bone is made up of protein fibres (called collagen) which give
elasticity and the vital mineral calcium, which makes bone hard
and rigid.

Osteoporotic bone cross-section

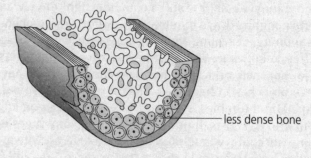

— less dense bone

Thinning is mainly due to loss of collagen, which removes calcium
with it. Both the hard dense bone and the more spongy springy
bone tissue are affected.

Figure 11

continue to grow in strength well into the mid-twenties. By then
peak bone mass is achieved and the skeleton becomes stronger
than at any other time during life. From that time up until the
age of about 35 bone formation is matched by bone breakdown
to achieve a steady status quo. After the age of 35, bone loss

increases as part of the natural ageing process and it is this, coupled with various factors which can decelerate or accelerate it, that determines a woman's risk of future fracture.

Women are certainly more at risk of developing osteoporosis than men. For a start they have smaller bones which are less dense, and at the time of the menopause relative oestrogen deficiency greatly accelerates bone loss. If women have low circulating levels of oestrogen when they are younger for any reason they are at special risk of brittle bone disease, and there are a number of situations which can bring this about. Regrettably, the majority of women never notice the changes which are occurring and the condition is without symptoms. For this reason osteoporosis has been described very appropriately as the silent epidemic.

The Size of the Problem

More than one third of adult women and a sixth of all men will suffer at least one osteoporotic fracture during their lifetime. In women over the age of 50 osteoporosis results in over 150,000 fractures per year in the UK. These statistics make bleak reading. Every year nearly 70,000 people suffer a hip fracture. Fifty per cent of them have their mobility severely impaired. Twenty per cent actually die within the first year after the fracture, and more than 20 per cent of orthopaedic hospital beds are taken up with hip fracture patients at any one time. Furthermore, hip fractures make up nearly 90 per cent of the annual £942 million bill that osteoporosis costs the NHS and Government, not to mention the misery and pain and loss of independence that arises for the patients themselves. Whilst hip fractures are relatively commonplace and much talked about, the problems associated with vertebral fractures are often underestimated. A third of these spinal fractures cause deformity and may result in a significant degree of back pain, both acute and chronic. The dowager's hump has already been described as has the loss of height. Other features include a protruding abdomen as the lumbar spine is pushed forward, impaired mobility, indigestion, difficulty in breathing, general poor health, loss of self-esteem and self-reliance and, inevitably, increased mortality. One of the commonest fractures of all, a wrist fracture known as a Colley's fracture, occurs following a simple fall on to the outstretched hand. If I had been paid £5 for every one of these I have re-set in Casualty departments I would by now be a rich man. Sixteen per cent of women aged 45 to 54 require hospitalisation following this wrist fracture, rising to 76 per cent of women over the age of 85. Extended periods of pain, swelling and circulatory disturbances of the affected hand can follow. Restriction of movement can last for well over a year following the fracture and many patients never regain function of the wrist properly without physiotherapy.

Who is at Risk?

The impact of the menopause on women's bones makes them far more likely than men to develop osteoporosis. There are other extraneous factors, some medical, some due to genetics and others associated with lifestyle which can affect a woman's chances of developing brittle bone disease.

Risk factors for osteoporosis

1. Lack of oestrogen caused by an early menopause, that is, before the age of 45.
2. Lack of oestrogen caused by having an early hysterectomy, that is, before the age of 45, especially when both ovaries are removed (oophorectomy).
3. Lack of oestrogen caused by a medical menopause as a result, for example, of chemotherapy or radiotherapy.
4. Lack of oestrogen due to missing periods for six months or more (other than during pregnancy) as a result of severe weight loss due to over-exercising or dieting.
5. Having a close family history of osteoporosis.
6. Smoking cigarettes.
7. Drinking excessive amounts of alcohol.

8. Taking high dose or long-term oral steroids, for example for asthma, arthritis or other inflammatory conditions.
9. Long-term immobility.
10. Not getting enough exercise generally.
11. Doing excessive amounts of exercise and losing too much weight.
12. Having an unbalanced diet, particularly if it is low in calcium.
13. Having other medical conditions, such as an overactive thyroid gland, diabetes, kidney and liver disorders, Cushing's Syndrome, Crohn's Disease or Coeliac Disease.
14. Being small and thin.

It is important to realise that it does not necessarily mean that if one or more of these risk factors apply to you that you will inevitably develop a fractured bone in the future and become disabled. All it means is that it becomes even more important that you do as much as you can to help yourself to prevent problems in the future, even if you have already been diagnosed as having osteoporosis.

How Do you Know if you are Developing Osteoporosis?

Osteoporosis is known as the silent epidemic because none of us can see or feel our bones becoming thinner and less strong. For many people the first sign that there is a problem comes when a bone is fractured, often in the wrist or the spine after a minor stumble or fall. Wrist fractures are especially common in women in their fifties but regrettably the medical profession lags behind recent scientific discoveries so that the opportunity is lost of identifying, among women who have already suffered such fractures, those who are at risk in the future. It is a matter of enormous regret that dramatic loss of height in women, due to crush or wedge fractures, is allowed to happen despite available treatment, especially as chronic pain can result. The simple truth is that there are now a number of methods of testing for osteoporosis and even of predicting to some extent who is at risk of future fractures. These tests can also determine the rate of bone loss in that individual and monitor the effect of treatment if the test is conducted at intervals of 12 to 24 months.

There are a number of available options. Standard x-rays of bone are not particularly useful because although they can show an existing fracture, osteoporosis itself only shows on an x-ray when at least 30 per cent of the bone density has already been lost. More sensitive tests are required. The gold standard test is a bone density scan otherwise known as a dual energy x-ray absorptiometry (DXA). This is currently the most accurate and reliable way of assessing the strength of bones and anybody's risk of a future fracture. It is a straightforward procedure using a very low dose of radiation, about one tenth of the dose used in a standard chest x-ray. The patient is asked to lie down on the machine for about 10 to 15 minutes whilst an x-ray arm passes over them to record an image of the spine and hip. In some clinics forearm machines are used which measure the density of bone at the wrist. Women having this test are asked to avoid wearing clothes with any metal buttons, studs or under-wiring as these can interfere with results.

The results reveal how any individual's bone density compares to the average bone density for someone of the same sex and age. It is bone mineral density (BMD) which is being measured and the results are reported as a percentage of the normal value, or as a 'standard deviation', in other words the number of units above or below the average for the population. In 1994 the World Health Organisation quantified osteoporosis as follows:

1. *Average bone mass:* within one standard deviation of average for young adults.
2. *Low bone mass (osteopenia):* between minus 1 and minus 2.5 standard deviations below this average.
3. *Osteoporosis:* below minus 2.5 standard deviations.
4. *Severe osteoporosis:* below minus 2.5 standard deviations plus one or more fractures.

By the same WHO criteria, for each reduction of one standard deviation the risk of fracture doubles. In other words, according to the above chart, a woman with osteoporosis has at least five times the average risk of having a fracture in the future. There are, however, some disadvantages involved in DXA scans, not least of which is the fact that access to them in some parts of Britain is very limited. The machines are expensive, skilled staff are required to operate them and the tests take some time. There are therefore other methods of assessment which are currently being looked into, including urine tests and ultrasound measurements. Computerised axial tomography (CAT scans) is another method of scanning bones but is less attractive as it delivers a greater dose of radiation and is also expensive. Bone marker tests on urine samples can be used in addition to DXA scans to monitor response to treatment. When bone is being resorbed by osteoclasts, fragments of collagen (the scaffolding cross links between bone particles) are released into the circulation and excreted by the kidneys into the urine where they can be measured. Where bone is being formed the proteins made by the osteoblast (osteocalcin) are released into the bloodstream and can also be measured in a blood sample. These markers reflect the rate of bone turnover and since we know that in post-menopausal women the higher the bone turnover the higher the rate of bone loss, doctors can accurately assess the state of play. Treatments for osteoporosis result in a large and rapid reduction in the bone turnover markers and therefore increasingly in the future we will almost certainly be using bone turnover markers and bone density measurements to monitor response to treatment. One such test is even available to the public in the form of a self-testing kit for use at home. While testing kits have a valuable role within specialist centres, the NOS, however, does not support their use among the general public at this time.

The other main method used to assess bone density is ultrasound. Here an electronic image of bone structure and mass is obtained by use of a portable machine directed at the heel bone. The technique is painless and at least in women over the age of

70 ultrasound testing appears to provide an accurate assessment of hip fracture risk. One remaining problem is that results obtained by using different methods cannot be compared with one another and even the same tests carried out on different machines do not bear accurate comparison. Because changes in bone turnover in response to treatment are not measured so accurately in heel testing, DXA scans still remain the best option available.

All these choices and all this technology may sound very confusing but the existence of choices in medical screening is actually a very welcome thing. It is a good idea to discuss your options with your GP to see what is appropriate and what is available locally. Being well informed is always helpful as it enables you to push more constructively for what you want – particularly if your GP's knowledge on the subject is rather out-of-date, which, regrettably, it sometimes may be.

Who, in Particular, Should Have a Scan

Like many screening procedures, bone scans have a limited ability to make accurate predictions about who is at risk of future fracture and who therefore requires treatment. If the whole population was screened many predictions would be incorrect, leading to unnecessary worry and inappropriate treatment. Some would even be given the all clear whereas in fact they might actually require therapy. So doctors have come to realise that bone scans are most reliable when they are carried out on women who are at high risk. Current UK Department of Health guidelines therefore recommend that doctors refer only women at high risk of osteoporosis for screening with DXA bone scans, and these include the following groups:

1. Women who have had a natural menopause or a surgical or medical menopause before the age of 45.
2. Women who have had a hysterectomy leaving one or both ovaries before the age of 45.

3. Women who have missed their periods for six months or more for reasons not including pregnancy.
4. Women who are post-menopausal with other risk factors for osteoporosis.
5. Women who have had previous osteoporotic fractures.
6. Women who lack hormones for chromosomal reasons.

All women fitting into the above groups are now recommended to have five-yearly NHS bone scans according to these guidelines. In reality the family doctor may decide on referring a patient directly for a scan or choose to refer in the first instance to a specialist consultant. Another option which may be taken is to prescribe hormone replacement therapy at the menopause for women who are keen on taking it, in which case a bone density scan may not be required as the therapy provides an excellent level of protection against osteoporosis in itself.

How to Prevent Osteoporosis

It is not always possible to avoid all the factors which can bring about osteoporosis. Nobody can avoid growing older and nobody can alter their family history. Women who are naturally slim and tall and who have other medical conditions, perhaps requiring steroids, or women who have had an early menopause cannot change these realities. But looking at the list of risk factors which make osteoporosis more likely there are definitely lifestyle factors that can be altered. Since smoking is a contributory factor, cutting down or preferably giving up altogether is an excellent move to make for all kinds of reasons. Cutting down on alcohol intake and enjoying regular exercise of a weight bearing nature pays enormous dividends too.

Dietary Measures

The mineral which is most essential for building and maintaining healthy bones is calcium, together with vitamin D, which is vital for calcium's absorption. Table 1 shows the recommended daily intake of calcium; Table 2 shows the best calcium-rich foods.

Table 1

Child 7–12 years old	800mg
Teenager 13–19 years old	1,000mg
Adult male	1,000mg
Women 20–45 years old	1,000mg
Pregnant and nursing women	1,200mg
Pregnant and nursing teenagers	1,500mg
Women over 45 years old	1,500mg
Women over 45 years old on HRT	1,000mg

Table 2

Full fat milk ⅓ pint	224mg
Semi-skimmed milk ⅓ pint	231mg
Skimmed milk ⅓ pint	235mg
Small pot of yoghurt	240mg
Small pot of low fat yoghurt 100g	160mg
Parmesan cheese 30g	360mg
Cheddar cheese 30g	216mg
Sardines (tinned) 100g	540mg
Spinach 100g	170mg
Tofu* 100g	1,450mg
2 slices of bread	40/75mg

* Different products can vary considerably

Good sources of vitamin D, essential for calcium absorption, can be found in cod liver oil, oily fish such as sardines, herring, salmon and tuna, liver, egg yolk and margarines. The human body can also make its own vitamin D as a result of exposure to ultraviolet light on the skin. Only 15 minutes a day outside is required during the summer months, although burning should always be avoided with the use of appropriate sunscreens. Other sources of calcium include green leafy vegetables, most nuts and seeds, and dried legumes such as beans, lentils and peas. The best source of calcium overall, however, as you can see from

Table 2 is soya bean curd in the form of tofu. Whilst an adequate intake of calcium is important, there are also elements in the diet which can rob the body of calcium and this includes too much saturated fat, excess salt and very high consumption of protein as well as of caffeine from tea, coffee and cola drinks. Smoking and drinking also interfere with the body's ability to absorb and use calcium.

Exercise

Exercise plays an important part in helping to reduce the risk of osteoporosis. Bone is a living tissue which responds to increases in loads and forces by growing stronger. Because it does this constantly anyway, exercise will only increase bone strength further if it increases the loading above normal levels. For this reason, weight bearing exercise such as jogging and brisk walking can increase bone density in the spine and hips, and arm loading exercises such as weight training can increase bone density in the wrist if a person is not used to doing these activities normally.

The ideal exercise to prevent osteoporosis is to perform short bursts of exercise including high impact. This creates a large force which peaks rapidly as, for example, in the heel strike when your leading foot hits the ground during jogging or skipping. A few jolts are enough. It has been estimated that running up an average flight of stairs provides ten jolts each time you go up and ten jolts each time you come down. Ten flights a day provides 100 jolts which is probably adequate, whereas half an hour's jogging provides as many as 2,000 jolts. Many will be relieved to hear that prolonged exercise does not necessarily stimulate bone strength very much further.

The important thing is to take up an exercise or activity that is compatible with your lifestyle and which you enjoy, and is effective for improving bone density. Remember that although swimming and cycling are wonderful forms of cardiovascular exercise, and are therefore particularly good in reducing the risk of heart disease, they are not weight bearing and therefore have little value in the prevention of osteoporosis. A variety of exercises and activities is therefore required for women after the menopause to stay in tip-top health generally. Remember not to rush into unaccustomed exercise too quickly as this can lead to injury and stiffness. A minor amount of stiffness on the other hand lets you know that you have pushed yourself a little harder than usual, which will bring about improvement.

Exercise needs to be taken regularly to be of benefit and it is something that needs to be incorporated into one's regular lifestyle and adopted permanently because once exercise stops any improvement will gradually wear off. On the other hand, avoid becoming an exercise addict. It is possible to exercise too much and reduce body weight excessively, leading to lower oestrogen levels and an acceleration of bone turnover. Recommended kinds of exercise include jumping and skipping, stair climbing, jogging, exercise to music classes, weight training and field sports, racquet sports or dancing.

Complementary Therapy

Complementary therapy is becoming increasingly popular at the beginning of the new millennium and although medical evidence is limited many women, after the menopause, find such therapies beneficial. Various massage techniques can stimulate the muscular skeletal system, ease out stiffness induced through exercise and bring about a feeling of wellbeing. Naturopathy can improve a woman's diet and provide healthy guidelines in terms of calcium and vitamin D supplementation. Exponents of manipulative medicine, osteopaths and chiropractors, can apply physical techniques to relieve pain and increase mobility, although both types of therapists can also advise on specific exercises. Teachers of the Alexander Technique can retrain people to adjust their posture and poise in order to minimise stresses and strains on the skeleton. Acupuncture, which works by altering the flow of energy around the body, has now been adopted by most NHS hospitals with a view to improving mobility and relieving pain. Provided a complementary therapist is properly qualified, has a good reputation and is registered with one of the national organisations, experimentation with such techniques can certainly do no harm.

Public Health Measures

For older people especially, strength training, balance and low impact aerobic exercise may reduce the risk of falls. Home visits to assess and, if necessary, modify environmental and personal risk factors can also be effective. The use of external hip protector pads has been shown to reduce hip fractures in older patients in institutional care who are at high risk of falling. Any use of hypnotics and antidepressants in such patients should be kept to a minimum but, when absolutely necessary, should be used with caution as their side effects are known to increase the risk of falls.

Medical Treatments

Calcium supplements have been shown to slow bone loss in post-menopausal women so if dietary calcium intake is inadequate, supplements in a daily dose of 1g or more of elemental calcium may be recommended. This, together with vitamin D in a dose of 400 to 800iu (international units) daily, may reduce fractures in older patients as shown in at least two recent medical trials.

The other important group of medicines available for use in osteoporosis, where HRT is not suitable, includes the biphosphonates. This group includes alendronate (Fosamax) and etidronate with calcium (Didronel PMO) and risedronate (Actonel). Alendronate is licensed for the prevention and treatment of corticosteroid-induced osteoporosis in men and women, and for the prevention of osteoporosis in post-menopausal women considered to be at risk of developing the disease. Editronate is licensed only for the treatment of osteoporosis in post-menopausal women. Both are capable of reducing vertebral fractures and reversing bone loss to a measurable degree, and there is some evidence that each can reduce the incidence of other fractures, too. Adverse effects, however, include gastro-intestinal upsets and headaches. Risedronate is licensed to reduce the risk of vertebral fractures in post-menopausal women with established osteoporosis (women who have had a fracture due to osteoporosis). It is also licensed for the prevention of osteoporosis in post-menopausal women with increased risk of osteoporosis, and to maintain or increase bone mass in post-menopausal women undergoing long-term high-dose corticosteroid treatments.

Hormone replacement therapy, however, remains the gold standard for the prevention and treatment of osteoporosis. When menopausal women start treatment with HRT, the density of their bone rises by between 5 per cent and 7 per cent in the first year of treatment and then appears to remain about the same whilst HRT is continued. It is thought that the risk of hip fracture is reduced by about 30 per cent and spinal fracture by about 50 per cent when treatment is continued for five years. Continuing to take HRT for ten years is calculated to reduce density loss by 10–15 per cent, which would otherwise result in a doubling of the risk of fracture. However, when hormone replacement therapy is discontinued bone loss starts again and some scientists believe that the bone loss occurs at an even quicker rate than it would have done before treatment. This translates into the rather worrying fact that ten years after stopping HRT women can be shown to have the same bone density and risk of later fractures as those women who never took HRT in the first place. This poses the important question to doctors that if a woman's risk is greatest 25 years after her natural menopause, when should she start to take HRT and for how long should she take it? The answer is that HRT should remain the mainstay of osteoporosis prevention but that patients should be aware that it must be taken long term for maximum benefit. HRT should be offered to women with an early natural menopause or a surgically or medically induced menopause, but for other women decisions should be made after discussion of the relative risks and benefits of HRT. Furthermore, if you have specific risk factors or personal preferences regarding treatment you may need to discuss in detail with your doctor the pros and cons of treatment before a decision is made.

Progesterone Skin Cream

Finally, on the subject of hormone replacement therapy, a brief word about natural progesterone skin cream as this continues to excite interest in Britain, particularly as an alternative to HRT. Claims have been made by Dr John Lee in America that these creams are effective in preventing post-menopausal bone loss and can actually increase lumbar spine bone density, but unfortunately his data does not satisfy scientific scrutiny. A two-year study at Southampton, carried out under the auspices of the National Osteoporosis Society, is currently underway but no data are yet available. The first placebo controlled study on the effect of the cream on bone mineral density was completed, however, in the USA but results after one year showed that the number of women who gained more than 1.2 per cent bone mineral density with the treatment was not significantly different to the number of women who achieved similar results but were not on the treatment (they were on the placebo). In other words, progesterone skin cream offered no therapeutic benefit. Interestingly, however, there was a significant improvement in the symptoms of hot flushes and night sweats in women using the active cream compared to those using the placebo.

Tibolone and Raloxifene

Two other alternatives to standard HRT are worth consideration. Tibolone has oestrogenic, progestogenic and weak androgenic properties and may be used for the prevention of osteoporosis at the licensed dose of 2.5mg daily. It significantly increases bone mineral density in the spine over a two-year period, but whether or not it helps to prevent fractures has not been conclusively proven. Raloxifene is a new type of medication known as a selective oestrogen receptor modulator, or 'SERM', which has oestrogen-like effects on bone but the opposite effects to oestrogen on the uterus and the breasts. At a dose of 60mg a day, it can be used for the treatment and prevention of vertebral fractures in post-menopausal women at increased risk of osteoporosis. It does not, however, relieve symptoms such as hot flushes and night sweats at the time of the menopause. Its place in future therapy for osteoporosis is unclear at the moment since, being relatively new, its long-term safety is yet to be established.

The Future

Very recently, the gene involved in the control of bone density was discovered. This bone mass gene was found to be altered in patients suffering from a rare bone growth disorder known as sclerosteosis, a disease that is the exact opposite of osteoporosis. Learning more about how this disease actually builds stronger, more dense bones could help researchers in the future to understand the type of treatment necessary to strengthen osteoporotic bones, and to work towards being able to reverse bone loss in people who are at risk of future fractures. The process, however, of bringing any drug to market is a lengthy one and will take time. But for those currently suffering from osteoporosis this is exciting news for the future.

CHAPTER 9

BREAST CANCER AND THE MENOPAUSE

Although nine out of ten breast lumps are benign, more women develop breast cancer than any other type of cancer, with about 30,000 new cases being diagnosed every year. The chance of developing breast cancer increases with age. It is very rare before the age of 30, the risk at the age of 25, for example, being just one in 200,000. The risk then begins to increase in incidence as a woman reaches her forties, rising to a risk of one in 200 at the age of 50 and then one in 30 at the age of 75. But despite widespread fear about breast cancer, there is no epidemic as such of this disease.

Keeping Breast Cancer in Perspective

To keep a sense of perspective about all this it is important to remember that the figure that is often bandied around (that one woman in 12 will develop the disease) actually refers to the risk that a female baby has at birth of developing breast cancer by the age of approximately 90. Whilst it is true that a woman's risk of developing breast cancer doubles every ten years, this age-related increase in incidence is true of many cancers and it does not take into account the fact that nine out of ten breast lumps are found to be benign, or the fact that many women, including those under the age of 50, are successfully diagnosed and treated. The fear has arisen that breast cancer is becoming much more common. Media scare campaigns have partly contributed. So much so that Professor Michael Baum, a leading cancer specialist, was reported in 1997 as saying, 'It is possible to have too much cancer awareness.' He was referring in particular to a breast cancer awareness month which took place in November

1996 during which publicity about breast cancer was everywhere in the media, from broadsheet newspapers to soap operas. Huge advertisements were featured on the London Underground warning women that one in 12 would develop breast cancer. Professor Baum commented, 'To describe the risk of developing breast cancer in one in 12 is true yet unhelpful. This applies to a cumulative risk for women who live to the age of 85. The incidence of breast cancer under the age of 30 is extremely rare and yet it is these women who are bombarded by breast cancer awareness campaigns and as a result grossly over-estimate their risk.' He went on to point out that, judging from discussion with his colleagues, no one of high rank had been consulted on this campaign.

At the same time, whilst keeping breast cancer in perspective is important, it is still good advice to remain 'breast aware' and to carry out regular checks on your own breasts from time to time in order to be able to notice any changes or alterations which are out of the ordinary for you. Along with screening, this is the best way of detecting and preventing problems in the future.

Causes of Breast Cancer

No one knows for certain what actually causes breast cancer although we are aware of factors which increase the risk. It is not easy to try to calculate a woman's personal level of risk because so many factors come into play. Most women have little or no control over most of the risk factors anyway. But any woman with more than an average level of risk can take advantage of screening programmes and visit the doctor quickly if a problem is suspected. Table 3 summarises breast cancer risk factors that have been identified to date.

Table 3

Increasing Age Breast cancer is more common in older age groups with the risk doubling every ten years.

Periods which start early and continue beyond the age of 55 These are linked with an increased risk. A late menopause is therefore a risk factor for breast cancer as it seems that women who have a menopause after the age of 55 have double the risk of developing breast cancer than women who have their menopause before 55. It is thought that this is due to the prolonged exposure of breast cells to a woman's natural oestrogen, as this hormone increases cell division and therefore the chance of cellular abnormality taking place, as well as the possibility of accelerating growth of abnormal cancer cells once they have taken hold.

Delayed Pregnancy Women who become pregnant only after the age of 30 or who never have children also seem to be at greater risk than women who have children much younger.

Breast-feeding Women who have breast-fed one or more children have a lower risk than women who have not.

Previous Benign Breast Lumps Some women who have benign breast lumps which are examined under the microscope and show cellular changes known as atypical hyperplasia may be at slightly more risk of developing breast cancer. They will need more frequent breast checks in future.

Being Overweight Being significantly overweight does seem to increase breast cancer risk. This is almost certainly due to a diet high in saturated fat.

Drinking and Smoking A high alcohol intake has been linked in some studies to a higher risk of breast cancer, and smoking may be associated with breast cancer as it is with other cancers, although no direct link has yet been shown.

The Oral Contraceptive Pill There is a very slightly increased risk for women whilst they are actually taking the pill although the risk is temporary and will disappear ten years after stopping the pill.

Hormone Replacement Therapy Initially, in the first ten years, the health benefits outweigh the slightly increased risk of breast cancer although thereafter the risk becomes more important. For a menopausal woman of 50, over the next 20 years she has a one in 22 chance of developing breast cancer, which increases to one in 20 if she takes hormone replacement therapy for ten years. If she continues to take HRT for 15 years the risk goes up to one in 17 or one in 18. Recent studies, however, have shown that HRT does not increase the risk of highly malignant breast cancer but does raise the risk of some uncommon forms of the disease that are slow growing and highly treatable. Some studies have not even established any link between oestrogen used after the menopause and breast cancer and, reassuringly, some doctors have conducted studies to show an association between HRT and a small reduction in breast cancer deaths rather than an increase. Indeed the Women's Health Concern charity news release made this very point in their October 1999 publication. So the decision about whether to keep taking HRT beyond ten years has to be an individual one based on the pros and cons for each individual woman.

Family History One in ten women who develop breast cancer inherit some form of genetic abnormality making them more vulnerable to the condition. The risk is increased if several members of a woman's family have or have had breast cancer. The same is true if she has relatives who develop breast cancer under the age of 50, or she has relatives who have had cancer in both breasts or who have had certain other types of cancer, notably cancer of the ovaries, colon or prostate, at a young age. The same genes may be responsible for such cancers. Whilst nobody yet knows how many breast cancer genes there may be, five have so far been discovered. About one in three cases of inherited breast cancer are considered to be due to an abnormality in a gene known as BRCA1 and the same number to another gene called BRCA2, with the other three genes and the ones yet undiscovered being responsible for the remainder. Testing for abnormal genes is currently available only in certain specialist centres, and before any woman can be offered a test it is necessary for doctors to show that somebody in the family who had breast cancer carried an abnormal gene. Once this has been established women can be offered the opportunity to see if they are carrying an abnormal gene themselves and may therefore be at increased risk. Those women who do carry an abnormal gene have between 60 per cent and 85 per cent chance of actually developing breast cancer at some time in their lives, and therefore they have the option of adjusting their lifestyle and taking other steps to reduce the risk of this cancer developing. Regular intensive screening is one method, a more drastic one being to opt for a double mastectomy with breast reconstruction; another option is to go into one of the current drug prevention research studies to see whether breast cancer can be prevented medically from developing.

The Diagnosis of Breast Cancer

The first sign that an abnormality may be present may be that the women herself notices a lump or a change in the breast or it may be something the GP notices, or maybe an abnormality is discovered during the course of a routine mammogram. Breast awareness is an important skill to develop so that any change in the normal shape, size or contour of the breast can be quickly reported. It is understandable that a woman will be very worried if she finds something out of the ordinary but the quicker she gets it properly examined and investigated the better. See Figure 12.

Specific Treatment

Once the investigations and assessments have been completed, the most appropriate treatment can be agreed between the doctors and the patient. Treatment might include surgery, radiotherapy, hormone therapy, chemotherapy or a combination of these, depending on the cancer itself and taking into account the individual circumstances and preferences. Sometimes treatment will involve just surgery, although radiotherapy is often added to act as an insurance against any spread of the cancer from the breast into the lymph glands under the arm. Drug therapy might also be used in order to mop up any undetected cancer cells which could have escaped into other parts of the body.

A Positive Outlook

Despite gloomy statistics and the common belief that breast cancer is becoming very much more widespread, it is worth reiterating that breast cancer is becoming a little bit, but in fact

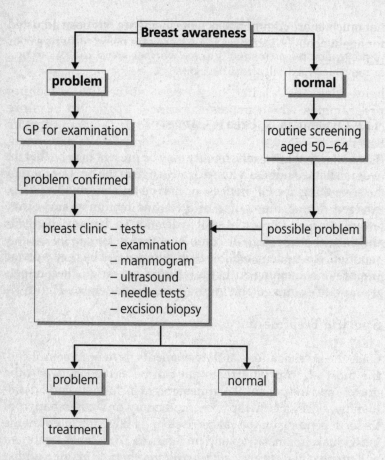

Breast awareness and routine screening remain the key to the detection of emerging problems leading to more detailed tests and early treatment of any disorder.

Figure 12

not much, more common. Once the incidence has been adjusted for age it actually increases by a mere one per cent per year or thereabouts. It is also worth bearing in mind that some of the increase could be accounted for by the fact that abnormalities are being detected earlier because of successful screening programmes which makes the cancer appear to be more common although it is just being detected earlier. Some doctors believe that if this is true we can look forward to a decrease in the incidence, or at least a levelling off of the incidence of breast cancer in the next few years, and in fact there is some early evidence that this is already beginning to happen. Of all cancers breast cancer is one of the most treatable and is associated with a high cure rate. Treatments overall for breast cancer are improving and so is survival. So despite the fact that increasing numbers of women develop breast cancer every year, the actual number of women who die from breast cancer is falling which proves the effectiveness of contemporary treatments.

CHAPTER 10

THE IMPORTANCE OF SCREENING TESTS

Screening tests are simple investigations carried out on a large number of apparently healthy people to separate those who may be developing a significant medical condition from those who are not. In recent years health care has advanced from merely providing a service for people who have become acutely ill to a system involved in preventative health measures also. Women in particular have welcomed screening procedures and as a result many hundreds of thousands of women have benefited. Some who had symptoms of one kind or another have been investigated and as a result of early diagnosis have been rendered free of their disorder. Others who had no symptoms whatsoever were made aware of a potential problem which they would otherwise not have known about for some time and have been spared suffering and hardship as a result. Many thousands of women have also had their lives saved by some types of screening, notably mammography and cervical smears. For this reason screening remains of essential importance in the maintenance of women's health. At around the time of the menopause there are many changes occurring within a woman's body which makes screening procedures of particular importance.

In previous chapters I have explored the nature and extent of many of the typical changes occurring at the menopause. Psychologically a woman can embark upon the menopause with very negative attitudes and unhelpful stereotypical ideas of how her life might be after her change. Even women who are upbeat about this time of their life, and who accept that the transition will lead to fresh challenges, can still harbour doubts and concerns about the future. In physical terms there are clearly major alterations occurring within a menopausal woman's body, not least of which are those affecting her reproductive system. Spiritually many women also need reassurance that their role within their family and within society as a whole is assured and will remain just as important as it has been before. It is likely that during this period of change most women will be visiting their doctor on an occasional basis anyway so it is a timely occasion to take advantage of any screening check-ups that are made available. It is logical that such screening procedures are taken up. Many disorders which develop unbeknown to women are age-related or associated with hormone fluctuations during the menopause and therefore become increasingly common at this time. This is why Well Woman Clinics can prove so useful.

Well Woman Clinics

These Well Woman Clinics are carried out by almost every NHS general practice in Britain and are run either by the practice nurse or by the family doctor or by a combination of both working in tandem. The actual list of tests and procedures carried out will vary from practice to practice but the vast majority would incorporate the following checks:

What do Well Woman Clinics have to offer

1. Opportunities to voice any general worries or concerns in women without symptoms.
2. Similar opportunities to talk about any actual symptoms.
3. Lifestyle questionnaire, including diet, exercise habits, domestic and work situation, alcohol consumption and smoking habits.
4. Baseline tests, including height and weight, blood pressure, urine analysis and blood sampling (for cholesterol, thyroid function, anaemia and diabetes).
5. A cervical smear.
6. An opportunity to discuss mammography or bone density scanning.

A Chance to Voice Your Concerns

Apart from anything else, a Well Woman Clinic or any clinic offering screening is an excellent opportunity for you to discuss any fears or anxieties you may have. It may well be that you are convinced that the menopause will change you in some terribly unattractive way and in this situation firm and positive reassurance can result in a much more constructive and helpful outlook. It sometimes means that symptoms relating to the menopause, of which you were not already aware, can be explained and treated. It also means that you can voice any niggling doubts about more sinister disorders such as cancer or degenerative diseases such as arthritis. These doubts may have arisen possibly because of a family history, or recent involvement with someone close who themselves suffered from such conditions, which may have resulted in a disproportionate degree of apprehension. Allowing you to talk about these fears so that they can be discussed in a cool and rational way may be very beneficial and may change the course of your post-menopausal experiences.

Screening for Women Who Have Symptoms

Many of the physical and psychological symptoms of the menopause may be readily remedied in simple and convenient ways. Providing you with the information and the wherewithal to deal with these symptoms can be enormously rewarding for nurses and doctors and patients alike. Two symptoms in particular are particularly relevant to screening procedures. The first relates to unusual patterns of vaginal bleeding and the second to abnormal changes within the breasts.

Any alteration in the usual menstrual pattern, any vaginal bleeding occurring more than six months after the last period, and any bleeding occurring between expected period times or after love-making should be regarded with suspicion and investigated further. Whilst stress, travel, changes in methods of contraception and even unsuspected pregnancy can lead to altered menstrual bleeding, bleeding occurring many months after the last period and bleeding after sexual intercourse might possibly be related to abnormalities in the lining of the womb or the cervix itself and require further examination. In particular cancer of the uterine lining or endometrium, as well as cancer of the cervix or ovaries, will need to be excluded.

The other vital symptom which can be investigated by further screening would be the development of a breast lump for the first time or an apparent change in a breast lump which has previously been noticed. In addition, any discharge or inversion of a nipple or any puckering of the skin over the breast needs to be explained so that any problem of a non-benign type can be excluded.

Routine Screening Questionnaire

A routine screening questionnaire to look at your lifestyle can be a convenient and useful method of making suggestions as to how you can best help yourself to make any changes necessary to ensure continued good health. Once the questionnaire has been completed some simple physical tests can be performed.

Height and weight can be measured and your Body Mass Index calculated. Knowing these parameters is important, because evidence suggests that middle-age spread after the menopause may be nature's way of protecting bones. An increase in fatty tissue after the menopause seems to help to maintain bone density, which can diminish if a strict diet is followed and results in significant weight loss. This is because the small amounts of female sex hormones produced by the adrenal gland and the post-menopausal ovaries find their way into the fat cells where they are transformed into oestrogens. When the weight in kilograms and the height in metres has been measured, the Body Mass Index can be calculated by dividing the weight by the square of the height, for example if the weight is 70kg and the height is 1.5m the BMI would be 70 divided by $1.5 \times 1.5 = 31.1$. The approximate BMI of 31 can be plotted on a simple chart (see page 69) to quickly determine whether a person may be considered underweight, normal, overweight or obese.

Blood pressure can be measured by the simple application of an inflatable cuff around the upper arm. Blood pressure is an important risk factor for the development of future heart disease, although it may also signify whether you are under undue stress or tension.

The provision of a urine sample is valuable whether you have any symptoms of urinary problems or not. Dipstick tests using special pads impregnated with certain chemicals can reveal the presence of abnormal constituents in the urine, such as protein, micro-organisms, blood or glucose, for example. Many an asymptomatic bladder infection, kidney disorder or diabetes has been diagnosed in this way.

A simple blood test can screen for four of the most common abnormalities in women of menopausal age. Measurements of the haemoglobin level can determine whether you have become anaemic, possibly as a result of heavy, irregular or more frequent periods leading up to the menopause. Thyroid function tests can reveal whether your thyroid gland, your body's thermostat, is underactive or overactive and perhaps instrumental in bringing about any inexplicable weight change. Cholesterol levels can also be assessed, revealing, in one in 500 cases, a totally unexpected hereditary condition known as hypercholesterolaemia, a condition closely associated with premature heart disease. Borderline to moderately elevated levels will require more frequent monitoring as these too can be associated with an increased vulnerability to circulatory problems, including heart attacks and strokes, unless they are adequately dealt with. Finally, the blood sugar level can reveal further evidence of any diabetes should it be present.

Dietary advice may be given to help keep weight gain to a minimum and to reduce the future risks of heart disease and diabetes.

An enquiry can also be made into levels of exercise taken, and encouragement given if this seems appropriate. In particular, the frequency and type of exercise can be advised with reiteration of the attendant benefits. These include lowering of the risk of heart attacks and strokes, reduction in levels of high blood pressure, reduction in circulating blood cholesterol, reduction in the risk of blood clots, reduction in weight, the prevention of osteoporosis, lessening the risk of premature death, reduction in the risk of diabetes, an improvement in mood swings, anxiety and depression, neutralisation of undue stress, an improved quality of sleep and the possibility of a diminution in the risk of certain cancers.

Tactful enquiry into occupational workloads, domestic pressures and personal relationships can provide an opportunity to share problems and, even if none are discovered, such an holistic approach to healthcare can significantly enhance the doctor–patient or nurse–patient relationship.

Long-term alcohol consumption is a standard question now in most insurance company medicals and most people are accustomed to being asked about it and understand the importance of keeping alcohol intake to within recommended maximum limits. It is not beyond the bounds of possibility that a nurse or doctor may even advise a patient to actually start enjoying a glass or two of wine a day as most evidence seems to point to the fact that this has a beneficial effect on health compared to being teetotal.

Finally, but by no means least important, a woman's smoking habits and the attendant risks this brings may be assessed. The purpose of such medical enquiry is not to censure or judge any person but there is no doubt that, medically speaking, giving up smoking or at least cutting down is the single most important measure anybody can take to improve their future health and well-being. There is now overwhelming evidence that smoking increases both heart disease and a number of degenerative and malignant conditions within the body, and can seriously curtail the quality and quantity of life. If a woman wishes to give up smoking but is finding it difficult the Well Woman Clinic is well placed to offer support, encouragement, motivation and further advice.

Cervical Smears

Whether carried out within the confines of a Well Woman Clinic or a routine cervical smear clinic, every woman who has ever been sexually active should certainly avail themselves of the opportunity to have this test carried out. The cervical smear test is a routine way of checking the health of the cervix by examining some of the cells from it to see if they show any signs of cancerous changes. The aim of the test is to obtain a sample of cells from the cervix, and in particular from the squamo-columnar junction. This area is where cells which line most of the vagina join together with the cells which line the neck of the womb, the cervix. This junction in particular is where pre-cancerous changes are most likely to develop. By gently wiping a specially shaped wooden spatula over the area, or using a small brush to collect cells from the canal of the cervix, a sample of these cells may be taken. If there are pre-cancerous changes in the cervix or if there are cancerous changes developing they will be visible in the cells collected by the smear test. The cells are then 'smeared' on to a glass microscope slide (hence the term cervical smear) and sent for examination under the microscope at a special laboratory, a procedure known as cytology. The cytologist observes various features of the cells and their nuclei and then, according to a set of carefully laid down criteria, decides which category the cells belong to: normal, pre-cancerous or cancerous.

Interpretation of Results

The results of the smear test largely decide what will happen next. If the cells are normal nothing will be required until the next screening smear test between three and five years hence. Different health authorities vary but by and large most routine tests are carried out between three and five years in Britain. If there is evidence of a virus infection (the human wart or papilloma virus) your doctor will discuss with you when the next test should be or if any further test or treatment is required. If, on the other hand, the cells in the smear tests show some pre-cancerous changes what happens next will depend on the degree of those changes and whether there were any other problems seen or felt in the cervix during the examination.

It is important to realise that pre-cancerous changes do not generally mean that cancer will result in the future. In the majority of cases pre-cancerous changes actually revert to normal again on their own, as witnessed by subsequent smears. But because of the fact that a small proportion of pre-cancerous changes will in fact lead to cancer, it always means that the woman concerned will require more frequent smear testing if the results are of a mild or moderate nature, although the doctor may recommend colposcopy if the changes are more severe. Colposcopy is a technique that allows examination of the cervix in much greater detail than with a speculum and also permits the doctor to use a substance that shows up abnormal areas and to take biopsies of these areas. It does not require any form of anaesthetic and clearly takes no part in a normal screening examination of menopausal women unless cervical smear test results warrant referral to a specialist. Routine smear tests should be carried out on all women who are sexually active, starting within a few years of becoming sexually active and then repeated every three to five years thereafter if the first result is normal. Ideally tests should continue until the age of 70 as the incidence of cervical cancer increases with age. If you have vaginal bleeding other than at the ordinary time of your menstrual period or if you have pain during love-making or discomfort inside the pelvic area then an immediate smear test may be appropriate even if the test has already been carried out within the three-year time scale.

Breast Screening

All women should become familiar with the concept of becoming breast aware. The Well Woman Clinic and other screening clinics can provide a wonderful opportunity to explain to women what this should mean. In the past it was hoped that if every woman carefully examined her breasts every month this would lead to earlier diagnosis of any suspicious lumps, and therefore save lives. This campaign was widely adopted and was called breast self-examination. It was later discovered that breast self-examination was not as useful as had first been hoped and now the emphasis is on breast awareness. The concept of this is that because everyone's breasts are so very different it is much easier for you yourself to notice any changes than it is for a stranger, including a doctor or nurse. You are therefore encouraged to check your breasts from time to time (but not obsessively) so that you become familiar with the usual appearances, contour, fluctuations and so on. This, it is hoped, will make you better able to seek medical advice if you notice any changes in either breast that are out of the ordinary. Leaflets may be provided at screening clinics to teach breast awareness and some clinics use synthetic models of a breast to help teach you what you are actually feeling for. Being breast aware involves the following:

How to be 'breast aware'

1. When preparing to have a bath or shower, stand in front of a mirror with your arms at your sides and look at both breasts in turn.

2. Now raise your arms above your head and look to see if there are any differences on each side.

3. Now put your hands on your hips and press inwards until your chest muscles tighten. Look carefully at your breasts again from every angle – from the underneath and sides – then lean forward and look at the shape of your breasts. Has anything changed? Now feel for any possible changes.

4. In the bath or shower use a soapy hand which will glide easily over the breast. For women with larger breasts, they may find this procedure easier if they lie flat on a bed.

5. Keep the fingers together and use the flat of the hand to move over the skin. Try not to squeeze or poke your breast tissue. Use the flat of the fingers to press the breasts gently but firmly, using the right hand to feel the left breast and the left hand to feel the right breast.

6. Feel every part of the breasts in quarter segments using the nipple as the centre point. In addition, check the nipple for any discharge, and the dark flat area around the nipple and under-

neath it for any lumps or bumps. Finally, feel up and in towards the armpit where the tail of the breast tissue lies. Do you notice anything new? These checks can be made once every month or two especially in the week after a period, or at the same time every calendar month if your periods have stopped. If any changes are discovered a woman should go and see her GP straight away. If a definite lump is confirmed, or if the doctor wants to have a specialist opinion, the woman is referred as swiftly as possible to a hospital breast clinic. Sometimes, if there is any reasonable doubt, the woman may be asked to come back for a follow-up examination perhaps after another period. If a woman is referred to a breast clinic, further investigations may be carried out, resulting in either reassurance or appropriate treatment. See Figure 12.

Mammography

A mammogram is a special kind of breast x-ray designed to reveal very early abnormalities of the breast long before you may become conscious of them. In Britain once you reach the age of 50 you will be invited by post to take part in the National Breast Screening Programme and re-invited once every three years until the age of 64. Mammography screening does not necessarily stop then, however, as further tests can be carried out if you wish it. Much current evidence suggests that this is in fact a good idea as breast cancer continues to increase in incidence with age.

The reason why women under the age of 50 are not routinely screened is firstly because breast cancer is less common in the younger age group and secondly because younger women's breasts are of a denser nature so that small abnormalities are not demonstrated so clearly. Lastly, health economists are quick to point out that screening of younger women is not cost-effective. There are one or two exceptions, however, namely those women who are considered to be at higher risk of developing breast cancer, perhaps because of a strong family history. But for the most part women over the age of 50, who are generally post-menopausal, are the most appropriate recipients of mammography. Prior to the procedure, you are asked to undress to the waist and to stand in front of the x-ray machine. Each breast is then positioned in turn between two perspex plates so that it is compressed and flattened. A brief pulse of x-rays then takes pictures of each breast. The test is slightly uncomfortable but the vast majority do not find it painful. In any event it only takes a few moments. Results normally come through within a fortnight and a small number of women are invited to return for a second test, either because of technical problems with the first test or because a suspicious area has shown up which requires further evaluation. It is important to realise that by no means does being asked to return quickly necessarily mean that you have cancer. If you find yourself in this position you will be fully informed as to the reasons why you are being screened again. Most people, men included, worry a lot that an abnormality will be discovered when they undergo a screening test. In fact only about 55 out of every 10,000 women screened by mammography are found to have a cancer, and of course their chances of having successful treatment and being cured are vastly improved because the abnormality has been detected at an earlier stage than would have occurred clinically. See Figure 13.

Doctors always do their best to ensure that the screening procedures which they recommend are in your best interests, and contrary to popular belief they have simply been made available to women through the National Health Service to prevent problems and to initiate treatment at a much earlier stage than would otherwise occur. Women understandably worry about problems and difficulties which have been encountered and widely reported in the media concerning cervical smears, but it is worth remembering that many thousands of lives have been saved as a result of cervical smear campaigns despite these difficulties. If you are undergoing mammography remember that although merely having a test initiates worry, the test does not last very long and you will be immensely relieved when the results prove negative. You may also worry that an abnormality may be missed despite having the test. In fact it is

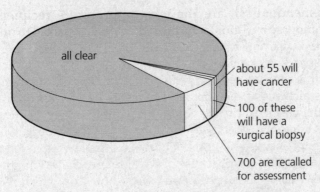

Out of 10,000 women having a mammogram, 700 will be recalled for assessment, of which 100 will have a surgical biopsy. Of these, about 45 will be clear and 55 will have cancers.

Figure 13 **Results of mammographies**

incredibly unlikely for an abnormality not to be discovered by mammography, particularly in women over the age of 50. Some women are in fact given a false positive result, suggesting initially that an abnormality is found but which proves to be completely benign after further tests. This only occurs, however, in about one in 100 women screened. Furthermore the x-rays used are not themselves harmful as the dose used is particularly low, and considering that four out of every ten lives lost to breast cancer can be prevented in women between the ages of 50 and 64 by breast screening, the advantages and benefits of submitting yourself for screening are enormous.

PART THREE

CHAPTER 11

PHYTOESTROGENS AND THE MENOPAUSE

Everywhere we look these days, whenever we open a newspaper or magazine, whenever we switch on the radio to hear a
programme about the menopause, we hear about phytoestrogens. Excited advocates talk about 'plant power' and the
'phyto revolution' and go on to make extraordinary claims about
the benefits of this natural alternative to hormone replacement
therapy. The publicity has been immense and the hype considerable. But is there any real substance behind these claims? Can
any health benefits be derived from certain plants, is this a particularly new phenomenon, and how much of it has been
exaggerated by a greedy and commercially motivated alternative health market raking in millions of pounds every year? Have
many women simply grasped the first hopeful straw they have
been offered once they have decided that traditional hormone
replacement therapy is not for them? Remember that only a
minority of post-menopausal women use HRT. Many doctors,
for one reason or another, remain reluctant to prescribe it and a
fair proportion of women who start taking HRT come off it and
discontinue treatment within the first six months because of side
effects which they associate with the product. Other women
simply should not take HRT for pre-existing medical reasons,
some do not want to and many do not need to. Any reasonable
healthy alternative then has its attractions.

Phytoestrogens of course are nothing new. Thousands of years
ago famous physicians employed foods and herbs to treat
medical conditions, long before vitamins and minerals had even
been identified. Hippocrates, the father of modern medicine,
lived and worked around 400 BC and wrote copiously about
the relationship between nutrition and health. Before him,

Dioscorides, the Greek physician, described some 600 plants which had therapeutic benefits. Plato and Pythagoras were keen on a vegetarian based diet for good health as was Galen, whose medical philosophies influenced Western medicine for the next 1,500 years. Since that time, whilst plant power has maintained a supportive role in health maintenance, in more recent times it has been eclipsed by the advent of more modern and much more powerful treatments, including antibiotics, steroids, immuno-suppressants and aseptic techniques in surgery, for example. Hormone replacement therapy, which was used for the first time just 60 years ago and which has been increasingly refined and rendered more sophisticated ever since, is yet another example. But all these potent modern medicines have their side effects and HRT, like all the others, has its critics. A renewed interest in phytoestrogens came about almost by accident, by observation of groups of animals whose diet was entirely plant-based. First of all farmers in Australia came to recognise a condition known as 'sheep infertility syndrome' where affected sheep were grazing on a specific species of clover. Due to adverse weather conditions affecting their normal feed, the sheep were grazed on a diet particularly rich in the clover Trifolium subteranneum which provided them with such high levels of biologically active phytoestrogens that it prevented the sheep ovulating and rendered them infertile. Similar reproductive failure was noticed in captive cheetahs being fed a commercially prepared feline diet with high levels of plant oestrogens. Close study of the cheetahs revealed changes in their bodies similar to those seen in women taking high dose oral contraceptives. Finally, in California, quails became sterile during particularly dry years; as their normal diet became scarce the alternative fodder for the quails had a higher than usual phytoestrogen content attendant on the drought conditions. These observations obviously got vets, doctors and scientists buzzing. If phytoestrogens could exert these powerful effects on animals, could similar effects be exerted on post-menopausal women?

In 1990, research published in the *British Medical Journal* and carried out by a group of Australian workers showed that menopausal women regularly consuming food and drink containing naturally occurring oestrogens, including soya products, organic linseed and red clover, were able to promote the same positive changes in the lining of the vagina as women taking hormone replacement therapy. Another study in 1992, this time published in the medical journal *The Lancet*, validated these previous findings. The study came to the conclusion that Japanese women did not seem to experience hot flushes and other menopausal symptoms because the typical Japanese diet contained foods very rich in plant oestrogens. Since then hundreds of scientific papers have been published confirming these results. Three fairly recent studies, one in England, one in North Carolina and one in Italy, all confirmed that when menopausal women enjoyed a diet rich in soya protein a significant reduction in hot flushes, by up to 50 per cent or more, was reported. The effect of phytoestrogen on the reduction of hot flushes and on beneficial changes to the vaginal lining stimulated work in other areas. In those countries featuring an Asian diet, the rate of hip fractures due to osteoporosis in women is only half that of the Western world. The incidence of breast cancer is lower (the ratio of breast cancer rates in England and Korea is 10 to 1); the incidence of coronary heart disease also shows vast differences, the ratio between the USA and Shanghai being 15 to 1. Also, Asian women are known to menstruate about every 31 days when the norm in the UK is about every 28 days. The effect of phytoestrogens is thought to lengthen the follicular phase of the menstrual cycle and delay the following period.

This is yet more evidence that phytoestrogens can have physiological effects in women. This has led to greater research efforts to determine whether phytoestrogens can influence other hormone dependent processes, such as cancer of the breast, prostate and uterus, heart disease and osteoporosis. Already, in the laboratory, several of these substances have been attributed anti-viral, anti-carcinogenic, anti-bacterial, anti-fungal and anti-oxidant properties so the relevance to this book of a diet rich in phytoestrogens is clear. But what exactly *are* phytoestrogens?

What are Phytoestrogens?

These are a group of substances found in plants. The phyto part of the name comes from the Greek word for plant. They are called oestrogens because they act like weaker versions of the human oestrogen sex hormones which help control female reproductive cycles. They are freely available from the diet. They are readily absorbed across the gut wall and undergo varying degrees of metabolism within the body. Both the parent compounds and their metabolites (the substances they are broken down into), many of which have enhanced biological activities, circulate freely within the blood and bodily tissues.

Phytoestrogens are present in nearly all plants in at least modest amounts, with some plants having particularly high levels. They are so ubiquitous in nature that they are common dietary components for most human beings. A mainly vegetarian diet can deliver blood levels of phytoestrogens several thousand times higher than that of the oestrogens made naturally within the body. So even though they are weak oestrogens their considerable presence in the diet undoubtedly makes a significant contribution to oestrogenic function in the body.

There are four main chemical classes of phytoestrogens. These are shown in Figure 14. The phenolic phytoestrogens (the flavonoids) are very prominent in the human diet and are present in all vegetables, fruits and cereals. They represent the largest single family of plant substances. Flavonoids are thought to act as natural fungicides, deterrents against insects and animals, regulators of plant hormones, and ultraviolet protectants. They all have a simple phenolic ring structure and are similar to steroidal hormones such as oestrogens and corticosteroids. Plants also contain a range of phytosterols which can be used as building blocks for the production of steroidal oestrogens within the body. Of all the flavonoids, the ones which have been most extensively studied are the isoflavones. Up to now over one thousand isoflavones have been identified in plants, mainly in members of the Leguminosae family. Of these, four have been shown to possess significant biological

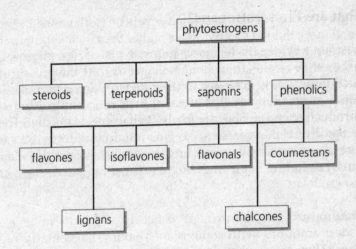

Figure 14 **The phytoestrogens**

oestrogenic activity, genistein, daidzein, formononetin and biochanin.

Genistein

This isoflavone is only found in soya and although it was identified as a plant oestrogen in 1966 it took over 20 years for its anti-cancer properties to be recognised by the medical profession. In post-menopausal women it seems to be able to block the effect of human oestrogen on breast cancer cells to some extent, therefore preventing their malignant proliferation. It appears to inhibit the activity of oncogenes, the genes that stimulate cancer and other enzymes which promote malignant change. It has also been shown to reverse the development of a cancer cell so that instead of becoming cancerous a cell changes back to being a normal cell again. Other studies have shown genistein to be able to block the blood supply to a cancerous tumour which results in it dying due to starvation. Professor Herman Adlercreutz, one of the main researchers in this area of medicine in the early 1990s, was able to show that Japanese men who consume soya products on a regular basis had levels of isoflavones in their blood more than a hundred times higher than their counterparts in Finland. Whilst the Japanese men had similar rates of prostate cancer, they tended to live much longer despite the presence of the cancer. The isoflavones in their diet appeared to make the cancer grow so slowly that it stopped the cancer spreading and did not affect the Japanese men's life expectancy. Other work has demonstrated that genistein plays an important part in reducing oestrogen deficiency symptoms occurring around the menopause, including hot flushes, night sweats, vaginal dryness and insomnia.

Daidzein

This is the other main isoflavone found in soya, and like genistein it also acts as an anti-cancer agent and an antioxidant, reducing the changes in the body which bring about degenerative diseases such as arthritis, heart disease and cataracts.

Formononetin and Biochanin

These two major oestrogenic isoflavones come mainly from red clover, chick peas, lentils and mung beans. Formononetin, a methylated daidzein, and biochanin, a methylated genistein, have unique effects on human physiology that are not shared by the non-methylated isoflavones genistein and daidzein found in soya. They would appear to be superior agents which may be more effective as anti-cancer compounds. They also appear to have a blood fat lowering effect which may account for the beneficial effect of phytoestrogens in the prevention of heart disease.

Lignans

Like soya products, lignans possess both weak oestrogenic and anti-oestrogenic qualities and are structurally similar to oestradiol. They come mainly from linseeds (flax seeds) and are converted by intestinal bacteria to hormone-like compounds.

Exciting new research is being conducted at this very moment to try to find out just how lignans modulate oestrogen function in the body and what their role in breast cancer prevention might be.

Phytoestrogens should not be confused with other kinds of damaging environmental oestrogens, the by-products of heavy industry such as that involved with pesticides, plastics and electrical transformer production. These xeno-estrogens or eco-estrogens, as they are sometimes called, have been incriminated in changing the sex of various forms of wildlife and to an increased risk of breast cancer in women. They have also been incriminated in falling sperm counts in men in recent years and other such horror stories. Because these synthetic xeno-estrogens are not broken down in the same way as naturally occurring oestrogens and tend to collect in the fatty tissues of the body, they are difficult to eradicate in nature and may be passed on from generation to generation. Phytoestrogens, on the other hand, are entirely natural and may be able to modulate abnormal fluctuations in oestrogen levels in the female body, whether they come from within or from the external environment. Many scientists are therefore taking an increasing interest in the benefits of phytoestrogens which include hormone regulation, correction of oestrogen deficiency symptoms in the menopause like hot flushes and night sweats, antioxidation to prevent the development of cancer, protection against osteoporosis, protection against heart disease, and in men the prevention of progressive prostate enlargement and prostatic cancer.

How do Phytoestrogens Work?

Phytoestrogens exert both oestrogenic and anti-oestrogenic effects on the body, depending on several factors including their concentration, the levels of oestrogens already in the body and a woman's individual characteristics and menopausal status. Isoflavones and their by-products are believed to be capable of preferentially activating different oestrogen receptors (see Figure 15). Phytoestrogens activate the beta receptors which are dominant in brain,

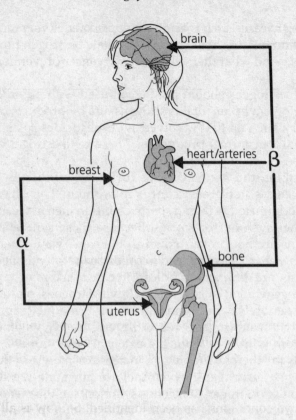

Figure 15 Locations of the α and the β oestrogen receptors

bone and heart tissues, but show little activity against the alpha receptors that are dominant in breast and uterine tissues. If this is the case they have much to offer menopausal women who do not want breast and uterine tissue stimulated but *do* require protection from heart disease, osteoporosis and various psychological symptoms (see Figure 16). The oestrogenic activity of isoflavones is relatively weak, however, of the order of a thousand times less than that of circulating oestradiol produced by the ovaries. Nevertheless, dietary isoflavones undergo varying degrees of metabolism at two sites in the body, in the liver and in the gut,

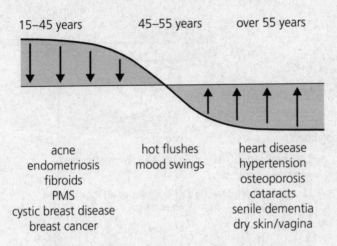

15–45 years   45–55 years   over 55 years

acne   hot flushes   heart disease
endometriosis   mood swings   hypertension
fibroids   osteoporosis
PMS   cataracts
cystic breast disease   senile dementia
breast cancer   dry skin/vagina

Figure 16 **Changing oestrogen levels throughout a woman's life**

through fermentation by bacteria. Some investigations have shown that once metabolised, they become between 10 and 1,000 times more potent than primary plant isoflavones, in which case a mechanism whereby they are capable of having such a profound effect in cancer prevention and the prevention of other degenerative conditions has been identified. So how is all this relevant to menopausal women?

Phytoestrogens and the Menopause

Figure 17 shows how an isoflavone can fit into the human oestrogen receptor site, wherever it may be located, and mimic the effects of oestradiol. But unlike oestradiol, phytoestrogens prefer to bind to the alpha receptor sites rather than the beta ones, leading to a smaller biological effect on the lining of the womb and the breast compared to the effect in other areas (see Figure 15). In high dosages isoflavones can have an 'oestro-genic' effect on the alpha receptor sites comparable with that of oestradiol. Yet, paradoxically, isoflavones can also display

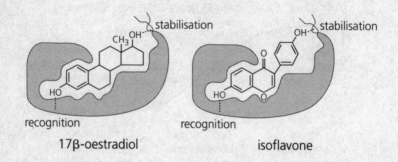

Figure 17 **The interaction of isoflavones and the human oestrogen receptor**

anti-oestrogenic activity. At low doses, by effectively sitting in the receptor site and exerting only a weak effect, isoflavones block the effect of a more potent oestrogen from reaching the receptor site, thereby reducing the total oestrogenic response. In this way isoflavones can act either as oestrogens or as anti-oestrogens depending upon the relative proportion of phytoestrogens and the body's own oestradiol. In pre-menopausal women, for example, where oestradiol levels are high, isoflavones act as antagonists or anti-oestrogens; in post-menopausal women, where oestradiol levels are low, they act as agonists or oestrogens. Some of the isoflavones are thought to display a particularly anti-oestrogenic effect similar to that of the synthetic anti-oestrogen drug, tamoxifen, which is used to treat breast cancer in post-menopausal women. In this way a balancing out of hormone fluctuation before and after the menopause can be achieved by enjoying a diet rich in phyto-estrogens (see Figure 18), and supporting this is increasing epidemiological evidence to show that many of the common degenerative diseases in developed countries, which are generally regarded predominantly as diseases of the Western world, are linked to low levels of isoflavones in the diet.

Figure 18

Average phytoestrogen content of food

Food	Daidzein (µg/g)	Genistein (µg/g)	Amount of food required to achieve 40 mg of phytoestrogen (g)
Tofu	76	166	165
Soy sauce	8	5	3,077
Soya milk	18	26	909
Soyabean sprouts	138	230	109
Soyabean, green	546	729	31
Tempeh	190	320	78
Soyabean paste	159	171	330
Miso paste	266	376	62
Miso paste (rice or barley)	79	260	118
Soya hot dog, tempeh burger	49	139	213

Are Phytoestrogens Safe?

Research continues all the time but before consumers rush out to embrace the new natural treatments for the menopause it is important for everyone to recognise the limitations of such treatments and to be alert for any potential risks. Since much of this scientific work remains in its infancy we cannot yet know everything about the safety profile of the phytoestrogens as many have only recently been discovered and their full effects have not yet been fully evaluated. This relative lack of clinical data must signal caution, specifically in relation to the possible risk of adverse effects, as well as enthusiasm regarding potential gains. Eating very high levels of some phytoestrogens may theoretically pose certain health risks. In laboratory experiments on animals, reproductive problems have been documented when phytoestrogen-rich plants have made up 100 per cent of the animals' diets. Human beings never eat an exclusive diet of such foodstuffs but those who eat uncooked soya or swallow large amounts of phytoestrogen pills as a natural therapy may be exposing themselves to some as yet unidentified health risk. Many natural compounds, especially hormones, can be potent and can have both good and bad health effects depending on how much of it accumulates in the body. These substances should always be used in moderation, therefore, to avoid any unforeseen or unwelcome health consequences. There must be a limit to the amount of phytoestrogens that will be beneficial to health and it is premature for anyone, especially pregnant women, to take phytoestrogen supplements until more is known. At a recent Menopause Society meeting in the USA, Kenneth Setchell of the Children's Hospital Medical Center in Cincinnati said that despite an explosion in research on phytoestrogens, the beneficial effects of soya are small when compared with conventional HRT. He also criticised some disreputable companies that are marketing soya supplements, and expressed concern that there appears to be very little scrutiny of supplements even though soya protein rich foods or supplements might, in theory, promote hormone dependent cancers in high risk groups.

In patients with breast cancer, the application of phytoestrogens as 'natural HRT' is becoming more widespread despite the fact that the safety profile has not yet been established. Phytoestrogens could very well turn out to be protective against the development and spread of breast cancer, but much may depend on whether breast cancer cells have receptors which are receptive to particular phytoestrogens and on the existing hormonal status of each individual woman. As the average Asian diet delivers between 50 and 100mg of isoflavones per day, it would appear reasonable not to exceed this dose. This coincides with a level that has been found to have a good therapeutic effect in several clinical trials and would therefore seem to be a reasonable compromise. Another potential safety factor worth considering is the genetic modification of soya products.

At the present time the desirability of genetically modified food remains controversial and many may wish to avoid it until such time as thorough tests rule out any possible long-term adverse effects. However, there are many companies who expressly do not employ genetically engineered soya in their products, including firms like Iceland, Holland and Barratt, Provamel, Waitrose and Wassen.

Phytoestrogen-rich Foods

Plant foods such as whole grains, dried beans and peas, beansprouts, seeds, vegetables and fruits contain phytoestrogens. Soya beans and soya based foods such as tofu contain some of the most active phytoestrogens.

Soya Beans

Soya beans can be eaten either fresh or dried. They may be added to stir-fry dishes, served as an hors d'oeuvre, as a side dish, or after cooking they may be served as soups, casseroles, curries, stews and burgers. Being fairly bland on their own, their flavour can be improved with the addition of herbs or spices in the cooking process. Soya flower may be added, along with linseeds, into bread recipes such as the Burgen loaf. Some brands of muesli contain soya flakes whilst soya cheese, soya cream, drinks, flour and grits are all available separately. Soya can also be eaten as a versatile meat substitute, and many more British women are now using soya milk in milkshakes, with cereals or added to sauces or soups. In the early days the beany taste made many of these milks unpalatable but the flavour has been improved immensely and such products continue to sell well. Miso is a fermented soya bean paste which usually has a smooth texture similar to that of peanut butter. It makes good soup but it is also excellent in marinade sauces and spreads. Tempeh is a fermented soya bean pâté which in flavour resembles strong mushrooms with a mild nutty, smokey taste. Its texture is chewy which makes it an ideal substitute for meat. Tofu, however, is

probably the best-known soya food amongst non-vegetarians
and has an almost sacred standing in Asian countries. It is bean
curd, similar in consistency to cheese, and it is an incredibly
versatile food to have in the kitchen. It has a very bland flavour
on its own but it easily absorbs the flavour of other food with
which it is being cooked, so for stews, kebabs, chillies and stir-
fries it is an excellent choice. Other soya products include
yoghurt, textured vegetarian protein, soya sauce, pasta and
protein isolate.

Linseeds

Fresh organic golden linseeds can be added to breakfast cereals
in a dose of, say, two tablespoons. They can also be sprinkled
over fruit salads, yoghurts, salads and bread mix. Alternatively
cold-pressed linseed oil can be taken in a dose of one tablespoon
per 45 kilos of body weight.

Legumes

The four major isoflavones can also be found in various legumes
including lentils, chick peas, mung beans and aduki beans. The
average phytoestrogen content of food can be seen in Figure 18,
and a good recommendation is that two servings of high
isoflavone products per day should be consumed in order to
obtain an intake sufficient to have a beneficial health effect. Some
women who are used to a Westernised diet may find any substantial modification of that diet difficult to attain, and
unpalatable anyway. Also, some soya milks are not as low in fat
as they could be and therefore have a potential to promote weight
gain when quantities sufficient to ensure a high isoflavone intake
are consumed. For that reason any of the new phytoestrogen-rich
supplements which may now be found in most chemists and
health-food shops may appear to offer a good alternative. The
diet which in total delivers between 50 and 100mg of isoflavones
per day is consistent with the isoflavone-rich Asian diet and
would seem a desirable target for which to aim.

Figure 19
Foods and herbs rich in phytoestrogens

alfalfa
aniseeds
apples
barley
black cohosh
broccoli
caraway seeds
carrots
cherries
chick peas
cinnamon
citrus fruits (including
    grapefruit, oranges,
    tomatoes)
clover seeds
cranberries
dahl beans
dong quai (Chines angelica)
elderflowers
fennel seeds
French beans
garlic
ginseng
hops
lentils
lime flowers
linseeds (flaxseed)

liquorice root
mung beans
mushrooms
oatmeal and oat bran
parsley root
peanuts
peas
plums
pomegranate
poppy seeds
potatoes
pumpkin seeds
red beans
red clover
red grape juice
red wine
rhubarb
rice
rye
sage
sarsaparilla
sesame seeds
soya beans (and other products)
sunflower seeds
tea
wheat
yeast

Overview

In all the clinical trials which have been conducted using phytoestrogen-rich foodstuffs, such as soya, red clover and cereals, it would seem that about two-thirds of women seem to have a satisfactory reduction in their menopausal symptoms if they consume sufficient of these products. But up to 30 per cent of any benefit obtained appeared to be due to the placebo effect;

in other words, when they were given a dummy foodstuff which was indistinguishable from the foodstuff containing the phyto-estrogens, they still appeared to benefit but purely from the expectation that they would. At the Sydney Menopause Centre and the Natural Therapies Unit at the Royal Hospital for Women in Sydney, New South Wales, no improvement in a post-menopausal woman's vaginal dryness was demonstrated, and any benefit in reducing cholesterol levels was thought to be independent of the isoflavones themselves. Nor, in the opinion of these researchers, was there any significant effect in the prevention of osteoporosis. So any woman wishing to try an isoflavone product for menopausal symptoms should be told that she has about a two out of three chance of improving her symptoms of hot flushes and night sweats over a two-month period. She may very well need a vaginal moisturiser or an oestrogen vaginal cream and she should certainly still have her bone density measured if she is in a high risk group for osteoporosis. Menopausal women will remain keen to try phytoestrogens as an alternative therapy to hormone replace-ment treatment, and because of this the medical profession and the scientific fraternity, often encouraged by women with an intense interest in the results, will continue to research these foodstuffs and phytoestrogen-rich supplements in order to be able to advise women more appropriately in the future.

CHAPTER 12

SELF-HELP AND COMPLEMENTARY THERAPIES

The majority of menopausal women will only ever experience mild to moderate symptoms. Many women, on the other hand, will suffer from severe symptoms and their lives can be made intolerable. What this actually means in terms of physical discomfort and change in the quality of their lives can be seen from the results of their menopause symptom assessment scale in Chapter 6. Whilst hormone replacement therapy is available to all, it will almost certainly not be appropriate for everybody and there is a small proportion of women who, for medical reasons, should certainly never take it. The later chapters of this book are devoted to the appropriate use of hormone replacement therapy, but for other women self-help measures, lifestyle changes and complementary therapies may be entirely sufficient to tide them over a temporary period in their life where they experience short-term symptoms of the menopause. These measures can also protect them from heart disease and osteo-porosis many years into the future. Broadly speaking, the simplest areas of your life to concentrate on in order to avoid post-menopausal problems include the food you eat, the exercise you take, keeping a positive mental attitude and taking steps to avoid any unnecessary stress or tension.

Nutritional Therapy

Nutritional therapy is usually referred to simply as 'healthy eating'. The word 'diet' has negative connotations of strict eating regimes, whereas nutritional therapy correctly implies a health benefit which can be achieved simply by changing the type of foodstuffs eaten rather than by cutting down on the amount. As women grow older their metabolic rate naturally slows by as much as 12 per cent by the mid-forties compared with 20 years earlier. This logically means that a woman's body needs fewer calories to generate the same amount of energy, but after a life-time's established eating patterns, it is difficult for many women to adjust their diet and eat less. A woman in her fifties with falling levels of oestrogen will also store any excess weight in the male pattern distribution on her body so that it tends to pile on around the waist and tummy. Since it is known that this pattern of weight distribution increases the risk of heart disease, nutritional adjustment is important, not only for reducing the risk but also to help women feel and look good. Sensible eating, however, is a habit which is initially hard to develop but which, once established, is fairly easy to maintain. Nobody should give up on dietary adjustment after a binge or an occasional gourmet meal, but yoyo dieting, where women continually put on lots of weight and then go on crash diets, is physically unhealthy and can be psychologically disastrous. Keeping your weight down also reduces the risk of diabetes and other medical disorders in the future. Here are some simple but important nutritional guidelines to keep you on the straight and narrow:

Choosing the right foods

- Choose, buy and prepare foods which are high in phyto-estrogens, such as soya products and legumes. Many plants contain molecules which are similar to, but weaker than, the oestrogen which is made in a woman's body but which also have oestrogen-like properties. The growing realisation that such foodstuffs can have a major role to play in the continued good health of post-menopausal women is such that Chapter 11 is entirely devoted to this subject.
- Go for low-fat dairy products, such as low-fat milk and low-fat cheeses, as these are low in calories yet are excellent sources of calcium for the maintenance of strong, healthy bones. Low-fat varieties in fact often contain slightly more calcium than the

full-fat varieties. Ideally, a woman should drink up to one pint of milk on a daily basis, but if this is not possible or palatable, calcium can be obtained from non-dairy sources including bony fish such as salmon and sardines. The sardines are ideal if the little bones are mashed up and consumed as well since these contain most of the calcium. Other sources of calcium include most green leafy vegetables but also peas, beans, lentils, nuts – especially Brazil nuts, almonds and cashews. Certain seeds like pumpkin, sunflower and sesame seeds are also excellent providers of calcium and other important minerals.

• Keep an eye on your fat intake. Only 30 per cent of the total calories that you eat every day should be in the form of fat. Most women would find that if they could cut their fat intake by about a quarter they would satisfy this criterion. For cooking avoid the use of butter, lard and hydrogenated vegetable oil, such as that found in shortening and hard margarines. It is better to use sunflower or sesame oil, or cold-pressed sunflower oil or olive oil instead.

• Go for particularly lean red meat or white meat. Some scientists believe that meat eaters have a lesser bone density than vegetarians as animal proteins can leach calcium and other minerals out of the bones, increasing the chances of osteoporosis. But lean red meat confers other dietary advantages and when taken every other day is fine, whilst white meat such as chicken or turkey is very low in fat and all fish can be happily substituted for either.

• Increase your intake of vegetables and fruit. Fruit is an excellent provider of fibre and because it contains fructose, a natural sugar, it is a satisfying substitute for refined sugar. Three portions of vegetables and a salad every day will provide a large amount of nutrients as well as extra roughage.

• Cut back on fast foods, junk foods and sugar. Refined sugar in sweets, chocolate, cakes, biscuits, jam, puddings, ice-cream and soft drinks can interfere with the absorption of essential minerals from the digestive system and lead to mood swings.

• Cut back on salt. Most adults consume far too much salt in their diet. This can lead to raised blood pressure, fluid retention and heart disease, as well as contributing to osteoporosis. Salt is already present naturally in food but vast quantities are added to processed and tinned foods before salt is added in cooking and then added again at the table. Avoiding too many salty foods, such as kippers, bacon and salted nuts, is a good idea. Substitute flavour enhancers include onion, garlic, herbs and a number of other spices, although very hot spices should be avoided if hot flushes are a problem.

- Try different cereals. Oats provide complex carbohydrate which provides sustained energy levels as well as fibre. Cereals rich in magnesium, such as buck wheat, barley, millet and rye, are also worth increasing in amount in your regular breakfasts.

- Drink plenty of water. Drinking up to three pints of pure water every day is healthy as it dilutes any toxins in the body and promotes their excretion, whilst reducing the risks of recurrent cystitis in susceptible women. It may also reduce headaches and dry skin caused by dehydration.

- Do not overdo the coffee and tea. Coffee is a potent stimulant of the heart and circulation as well as the nervous system, and can bring about dehydration. Many women working in offices during the week are tempted by plentiful supplies of free coffee and drink up to seven or eight cups of tea or coffee every day. It is enjoyable as a social break from work and also livens people up, making them more alert and better able to concentrate. However, come Saturday morning, when the caffeine intake dramatically falls, headaches and migraines caused by caffeine withdrawal are commonplace. Instead try decaffeinated varieties of coffee, or tea substitutes. Fennel, ginseng tea or other herbal alternatives are becoming increasingly popular. Even fizzy soft drinks can contain high quantities of caffeine, as well as phosphates and huge quantities of sugar and additives. Go instead for natural fruit juice based drinks or pure mineral water.

- Healthy snacks. Avoid hunger pangs, which can lead to bingeing, by keeping items like dried fruit or nuts and raisins in your handbag. Maintaining constant blood sugar levels reduces the risk of giving in to the craving for a large bar of chocolate.

Nutritional Supplements

Whilst following the above guidelines will help to provide most essential nutrients in the diet, the particular demands of the menopause can make specific nutritional supplements useful in banishing troublesome symptoms. Scientific interest is growing in 'sub-clinical nutritional deficiency' which means that although no measurable deficiency can be demonstrated within the body, supplementation can result in an improvement in symptoms and an enhancement of general well-being. Some experts believe, for example, that taking extra antioxidant vitamins such as A, C and E can lead to a reduction in degenerative diseases like arthritis, heart disease and possibly even cancer. Vitamins and minerals which are thought to be especially useful during and after the menopause can be seen in the box below.

Recommended vitamins and minerals

Calcium
Food sources: Dairy products including milk, cheese, yoghurt, bread especially white, sardines, green leafy vegetables, beans.
Function: For strong teeth and bones, normal nerve and muscle function, prevention of osteoporosis.
Symptoms of deficiency: None until it is too late, then osteoporotic fractures of hip, spine or wrist, back pain and loss of height.
Who needs it most: Women with early menopause, low levels of exercise, heavy drinkers, smokers, low dairy consumers.

Iron
Food sources: Red meat, eggs, fortified cereals, nuts, whole grains.
Function: Allows red blood cells to carry oxygen. Energy provision in the body.
Symptoms of deficiency: Fatigue, lethargy, lack of energy, depression, sore tongue, cracking at corners of the mouth, digestive problems.
Who needs it most: Women with heavy periods, vegans or vegetarians, heavy caffeine drinkers.

Magnesium

Food sources: Green vegetables, brazil and almond nuts, whole grains.

Function: Important in energy regulation within body and for healthy nerves and muscles.

Symptoms of deficiency: Mood swings, muscle cramp, depression, lack of energy, nausea, loss of appetite.

Who needs it most: Women with mood swings, irritability, fatigue, women who take diuretics, heavy drinkers.

Zinc

Food sources: Meat, legumes, peas, beans, nuts, lentils, whole grains.

Function: Good immune function, normal growth, hormone provision and reproductive health.

Symptoms of deficiency: Skin problems such as acne, recurrent infections, infertility, eczema, dry skin.

Who needs it most: Vegetarians, heavy caffeine drinkers, heavy alcohol drinkers, women on diuretics.

B group vitamins

Food sources: Meat, fish, nuts, whole grains, fortified cereals.

Function: Regulates protein use within the body, controls mood and behaviour, affects hormone metabolism, health of nerves and muscles.

Symptoms of deficiency: Anaemia, depression, anxiety, lack of appetite, nausea, insomnia.

Who needs it most: Heavy smokers, fast food fans, heavy drinkers, those with high sugar intake.

Vitamin C

Food sources: Most fruit and vegetables.

Function: Healing and repair of tissues, and production of certain hormones.

Symptoms of deficiency: Recurrent infections, lethargy, depression.

Who needs it most: Smokers especially.

Vitamin D

Food sources: Fatty fish such as halibut and mackerel, margarines.

Function: Essential for calcium absorption.

Symptoms of deficiency: Osteoporotic fractures later in life.

Who needs it most: Women on a poor diet, vegans, women
never exposed to sunlight.
Vitamin E
Food sources: Unrefined corn oil, sunflower seeds, peanuts,
sesame seeds, beans, wheat germ.
Function:Antioxidant protects cells from damage, prevents
blood clots, helps circulation.
Symptoms of deficiency: Lack of sex drive, exhaustion after light
exercise, easy bruising, loss of muscle tone, varicose veins.
Who needs it most: Fast food fans, those with poor diet.
Omega 3 Fatty Acids
Food sources: Cod liver oil, mackerel, herring.
Function: Controls inflammation.
Symptoms of deficiency: None obvious.
Who needs it most: Those on a poor diet.
Omega 6 Fatty Acids
Food sources: Many nuts and seeds, sunflower, safflower and
corn oil, green vegetables.
Function: Controls inflammation, keeps nervous system, skin
and blood vessels healthy.
Symptoms of deficiency: Severe eczema, PMS symptoms, breast
tenderness, mood swings.
Who needs it most: Those on a poor diet, diabetics and drinkers.

By understanding the nutritional content of foods, and with
reference to statutory labelling on foodstuffs, it should be easier
these days to select items of shopping which contain maximum
amounts of the nutrients required. Herbal supplements may
provide additional benefits and these are discussed on page 222.

Food Intolerance

A quick word about food intolerance. Unlike true clinical food
allergy (which results in an itchy blotchy skin rash, and possibly
even swelling of the lips and tongue, and breathing difficulties,
immediately after eating certain foods like strawberries, eggs or
peanuts), food *intolerance* is a more subtle and gradual reaction

to certain elements in food, resulting in symptoms such as behavioural changes or weight gain. There is increasing scientific interest in this phenomenon as a possible cause of some menopausal symptoms, and allergists, clinical ecologists and many complementary practitioners are convinced of a link although conventional doctors still remain sceptical. To keep things in perspective, research has shown that a small number of women, about 5 per cent in fact, can produce antibodies to certain foods. This can be short-lived and temporary or possibly life-long but amongst the potential food culprits, wheat and dairy products are amongst the most common. Symptoms such as mood swings, irritability, abdominal bloating, constipation, diarrhoea, joint pain, excessive wind, irritable bowel syndrome, tiredness and depression have all been laid at their door. Other foodstuffs incriminated include oats, rye and barley. The advice given is often confusing and it is not easy to prove whether a woman may or may not be sensitive to these elements in her diet. Finding out is likely to take at least six weeks, probably longer. The person being investigated has to exclude each suspected foodstuff totally from her diet and then six weeks later, if she feels that her symptoms have eased, she then gradually reintroduces it. If no sensitivity reaction to the first foodstuff occurs, another is then chosen and the process is repeated. There is no point at all excluding more than one foodstuff at a time because if a reaction does occur it will be impossible to know which one has caused it. The aim of this process is to identify which foods lead to symptoms so that the troublesome ones can be avoided in the future. Avoiding such foods can be difficult but it is certainly not impossible. Chemists, health food shops and many supermarkets now stock alternative grain products, for example, EnerG white or brown rice bread, Glutafin wheat-free bread and rolls, and Glutano flat bread, crackers and rice cakes. Alternative grain pastas are in plentiful supply, and as a breakfast cereal any rice or corn cereal, including rice crispies and cornflakes, are unlikely to cause problems of food intolerance.

Exercise

Taking regular exercise is just as important as eating healthily. People who exercise regularly are generally more in tune with their bodies and how they feel and function. They are likely to be more aware of any muscle tension, stiffness and loss of movement when exercise has not been taken for a while. People who are fitter through having taken regular activity often report the ability to think faster and more clearly. They feel better in themselves and have sharper, more acute reflexes. In fact they often feel so good they may be tempted to exercise too much. Some people spend inordinate amounts of time in the gym at the expense of their work and social life. This is because chemical neurotransmitters in the brain called endorphins, which are produced as a result of exercise, act like natural opiates in the brain. They give the person a 'buzz' and a wonderful sense of euphoria. But whilst addiction to exercise may be undesirable, appropriate levels of exercise are incredibly beneficial. Just look at the following list of advantages that regular moderate exercise can confer.

The benefits of exercise

1. Lowers the risk of heart attacks and strokes.
2. Lowers blood pressure.
3. Lowers cholesterol.
4. Reduces the risk of blood clots.
5. Keeps the weight down.
6. Prevents brittle bone disease (osteoporosis).
7. Lessens the risk of premature death.
8. Reduces the risk of diabetes.
9. Improves mood.
10. Reduces anxiety, depression and stress.
11. Improves quality of sleep.
12. May lessen the risk of certain cancers.

Different kinds of exercise may be better for different situations. For fitness and stamina, three or four 20-minute aerobic episodes of exercise every week are of maximum benefit. But for stress and tension based on anger, and for tension caused by frustration and rage, more vigorous exercise such as a hard session on the squash court or a cross-country run, kick-boxing or a work-out in the gym might be preferable. On the other hand, if the stress is caused by bereavement or from a relationship break-up then the person needs nurturing and comfort, and the body is more in need of tender loving care. Some long warm baths, gentle stretching, yoga, long walks in the fresh air and massages are more likely to be helpful. For depression, activity incorporating social involvement such as class work-outs, running groups and dancing are recommended. For anxiety, any exercise which uses up the stress hormones noradrenaline and adrenaline are useful, so cycling, jogging, aerobics classes or swimming can restore a sense of self-worth and calm. For the prevention of osteoporosis, weight-bearing exercise is the kind of activity which confers the most benefit. Brisk walking, jogging, skipping, high impact aerobics or simply going up and down a flight of stairs twenty or thirty times a day provides great advantages.

There are many different kinds of physical activity to choose from but provided a woman makes a decision to become more active every day it really does not matter what type of exercise she takes. Dancing is pleasant, but even allowing time to walk to the next but one bus stop, or parking the car further away from the supermarket so a benefit is gained from the additional walking, is worthwhile. Remember, however, that exercise should never be associated with torture or discomfort. It should always be fun and it should always make you feel good. Whatever it is you decide to do in the way of physical activity, remember these five essential guidelines:

1. Before starting, warm up for at least five minutes with stretching exercises and jumping on the spot.

2. Don't go at it like a bull in a china shop, build up your fitness slowly and make sure you exercise within the limits of your comfort. In time you will be able to do more and more.
3. When you feel excessively tired stop and rest, your body is telling you something.
4. Cool down again after stopping the exercise and stretch to avoid stiffness later.
5. Aim for a pace which keeps you moderately puffed and try to do both aerobic work and light weight work. Three times a week for about 20 minutes is ideal.

Positive Thinking

Contrary to popular belief, the menopause need not be that difficult time in a woman's life which she must simply grin and bear. Chapters 3 and 4 are packed with suggestions and specific treatments for physical and psychological symptoms which may arise during the menopause, but keeping mentally active and enjoying new friendships and interests, as well as maintaining personal relationships, is just as important. Throughout our lives our relationships with others, including our partners and close family, continue to develop and change. So rather than being aware of the empty nest left when children grow up and leave home, try to be more conscious of the freedom to explore new avenues which the menopause brings.

The stress involved in living in this new millennium can be difficult to manage, especially for women pulled in different directions such as working in a busy job as well as perhaps caring for elderly relatives. It is not easy to make provision to find time for yourself. But many surveys show that satisfaction in relationships which have survived to this point can blossom again. Many post-menopausal women and their partners actually seem to rediscover each other as individuals once more. For those couples who wish to continue to be sexually active, the physical problems brought about by relative oestrogen deficiency should be fairly straightforward to overcome. Vaginal dryness can be treated with extra lubrication in the form of Replens, KY Jelly or Senselle, although sometimes an HRT vaginal cream provides a more appropriate solution. Even libido can be enhanced if there is a wish for it, with various hormonal and non-hormonal preparations (see Chapter 5). Should a woman feel despondent about the changes she undergoes at the menopause, rather than feel unloved and as if nobody understands, taking the opportunity to share any concerns and anxieties can reap amazing dividends. It is vital to dismiss depressive thoughts and to deal with any anxiety and there are always professional people on hand who can advise, encourage, motivate and support even if your own partner is no longer there. Even for women who do find themselves alone and isolated it is always worth remembering that. Being on your own in later life can actually be very rewarding, sometimes more so than being caught in a loveless relationship. But an effort has to be made to keep socially active, to maintain closeness to good friends and to stay in touch with caring relatives. To any woman feeling emotionally vulnerable at the time of her menopause I would say the following:

- Plan new interests and ambitions. You spent years looking after other people's needs, it is high time to put yourself number one for a change.
- Plan some personal time for yourself each day and make space for reading, doing crosswords or listening to soothing relaxing music. My own CD *Music for Wellbeing* incorporates four specific relaxation programmes accompanied by some of the world's most relaxing classical melodies, together with some ethereal and imaginative new world music.
- Treat yourself with rewards and thank yous for what you have achieved.
- Think about travelling and going away, in addition to taking normal holidays, and plan for a weekend away from time to time.
- By all means indulge in some recreational shopping, but do not forget to keep an eye on the bank account.

Anything that gets your brain working and keeps you mentally alert is good and if you have the time think about joining an evening class, a local club or perhaps even taking up a university degree. Volunteer work for a favourite charity or support group can also be therapeutic and rewarding in the long term. Part of thinking positively involves changing the way you think about life so that you approach it in a more constructive fashion. To do this count up how many negative and unhelpful thoughts you have every day and how much of the day was taken up with them. Next work out some more positive responses that you could have substituted for each unhelpful thought so that you are seeing each problem in a different light. Then practise those positive thoughts and use them for each similar situation in the future. Ask yourself in any given situation whether your thoughts relate to the facts. If you tend to dismiss your own efforts and minimise them, your high level of self-criticism will begin to depress you. If, however, you concentrate on what you have achieved, you will feel better about yourself in the long term whilst becoming aware of how damaging those previous negative thoughts were becoming. Thinking positively gives you a sense of control in your life, of achievement and satisfaction. It motivates you, helps you concentrate and is picked up by people around you. So whenever you are tempted to think negatively remember that your unhelpful thoughts are not borne out by the true facts. You are jumping to conclusions. There are other ways of looking at any situation and there is a good side to most things. Do not let your unhelpful thoughts hinder you and hold you back. Stop thinking in terms of black and white, and that just because one thing goes wrong it changes everything else. Remember that you have strengths as well as weaknesses and try to praise rather than blame yourself. Do not be prepared to shoulder all the responsibility when things go wrong and remember that perfection is rare. It is terribly easy to allow things to get out of proportion, but trivial problems are never disasters.

So, have you got the message? Think positively!

Avoiding Unnecessary Stress

In this twenty-first century, the pace of life has become ever faster and more fraught. Everywhere we look we seem to find yet more sources of stress. It has become part of the fabric of modern existence. It is now something we live and breathe. Despite its potential for progress through understanding, co-operation and love, this is an increasingly overcrowded world facing more competition, selfishness and hostility at every turn. As a GP I see the effects of excess stress in my surgery on a daily if not hourly basis. I see high blood pressure, heart attacks, panic attacks and depression. I see irritable bowel syndrome, insomnia and migraine. I even see relatively new conditions affecting adults and children alike which are inextricably bound up with stress. Almost every patient who consults me is suffering from a condition that is at least in part exacerbated by the pressures, tensions and hassles of daily existence. Even the 50 per cent of people who do not acknowledge it in research surveys are detrimentally affected by subconscious stress.

Women in their peri-menopause and beyond are no exception. Often the fluctuations in their hormone levels, and the combination of physical and psychological symptoms, may contribute in making them even more vulnerable to tensions and pressures in their lives. This is a situation they do not want and do not need, and luckily there are many positive steps that can be taken to avoid them.

Assessing Life Events and Stresses

There are lots of little things we can all do to reduce pressure on ourselves. The first thing is to add up all the current stresses that exist in our lives at the present time following these simple steps.

1. Make a list of all your various sources of stress and how persistent they have been.
2. Arrange your list under various headings, such as trivial and serious, remembering that lots of little irritations and

niggles can be more upsetting than one single major difficulty.
3. Sort your list out again into the stresses that have immediate practical solutions, those that will get better in their own time and those that you simply cannot change no matter what you do.
4. Try to stop worrying about the stresses that do not have an obvious practical solution.
5. Start working on the stresses you feel can be changed. It is worth trying out possible solutions and seeing how you get on.

Tackling sources of stress may mean upsetting other people but quite possibly you have been putting yourself out for others for far too long and now it is time to put yourself first. Take a look at the 20-point questionnaire below to work out how stressful your lifestyle may be and to what extent it is contributing to any tension. Award yourself a point from one to ten. For example on the first statement, if you eat saturated fat at every meal every day give yourself 10 points, but if you eat it only occasionally, award yourself one point. Then do the same for all 20 statements.

Questionnaire: How Stressful is Your Lifestyle?

1	I keep my saturated fat intake to a minimum	1 2 3 4 5 6 7 8 9 10	I eat fatty food at most meals
2	I choose foods rich in fibre	1 2 3 4 5 6 7 8 9 10	I go for fast food generally
3	I make a point of drinking plenty of water	1 2 3 4 5 6 7 8 9 10	I never drink just water
4	I generally eat breakfast	1 2 3 4 5 6 7 8 9 10	I usually skip breakfast
5	I always have fresh fruit and vegetables at home	1 2 3 4 5 6 7 8 9 10	Most fruit and vegetables I eat are tinned

6	I hardly ever miss meals	1 2 3 4 5 6 7 8 9 10	I often miss meals
7	I take a multivitamin supplement most days	1 2 3 4 5 6 7 8 9 10	I never waste money on vitamins
8	I avoid too many strong, caffeinated drinks	1 2 3 4 5 6 7 8 9 10	I need strong coffee and other drinks to wake me up
9	I drink within the 'safe' recommended limits for alcohol	1 2 3 4 5 6 7 8 9 10	I regularly exceed the 'safe' recommended alcohol limits
10	I never binge on alcohol and get 'legless'	1 2 3 4 5 6 7 8 9 10	I often sink a few drinks too many and suffer hangovers
11	I never drink every day	1 2 3 4 5 6 7 8 9 10	I always drink every day
12	I do not miss a drink if I do not have one	1 2 3 4 5 6 7 8 9 10	I really need and crave a drink most days
13	I do not smoke, and never have done	1 2 3 4 5 6 7 8 9 10	I regularly smoke
14	None of my family and few of my friends smoke	1 2 3 4 5 6 7 8 9 10	I'm surrounded by other people who smoke
15	I exercise for at least half an hour three times a week	1 2 3 4 5 6 7 8 9 10	I last exercised when I left school
16	I'd rather walk up two flights of stairs than take the lift	1 2 3 4 5 6 7 8 9 10	I'll always take the lift if it's there

17	My work entails a fair amount of physical exercise	1 2 3 4 5 6 7 8 9 10	My job is sedentary
18	My weight is just right for my height	1 2 3 4 5 6 7 8 9 10	I'm very overweight for my height
19	I enjoy a regular sleep routine	1 2 3 4 5 6 7 8 9 10	I grab some sleep when I'm not burning the candle at both ends
20	I make exercise a priority and do it even if I'm tired mentally	1 2 3 4 5 6 7 8 9 10	I'll always put off exercise if I'm too tired

Self-assessment

The higher your score in this questionnaire the less healthy a lifestyle you are leading. Each high-scoring answer increases your vulnerability to stress, even though you may be adopting certain habits in the mistaken belief that they are helping you cope with stress.

Above 140 points

With the lifestyle you are leading, you are heading for an early grave! You may not be aware of it now, but the way you are living will be taking its toll on you. Many of the early warning signs of stress which you will exhibit are being made worse by what you are doing to yourself. Take steps to change things now.

90–140 points

This is better, but there is still no room for complacency. Any increase in unfavourable life events, or in stresses at work or at home, and your lifestyle could easily take an unhealthy turn for the worse. Get into regular healthy habits and make exercise and leisure a priority.

Below 90 points
Well done! Your lifestyle is a healthy one and gives you the best possible chance of being able to cope with all the hassles and pressures of life to your best advantage. You will also be more in tune with your body and be able to react more quickly if your stress levels build up.

If we are honest most of us will admit to leading fairly hectic and stressful lifestyles. Though stress in itself is seldom the sole cause of ill health, it can certainly contribute to a far ranging catalogue of disorders. These include fatigue, anxiety and depression, along with heart disease, palpitations and breathlessness, right through to digestive complaints, skin problems and irrational and uncontrollable anger. The inexorable build up of tension within us may express itself in a number of ways. Incredibly you may not even be aware that you too are becoming yet another victim of unremitting stress. Could you be drinking or smoking more than usual? Have you lost your appetite or gained weight because you have been eating for emotional comfort? Are you constantly irritated, impatient or finding it hard to concentrate and make decisions? If so you may be more wound up than you realised. And if you sometimes feel unable to cope and, for example, cry at the least little thing and are constantly tired for no good reason, you need to learn to let go of tension much more urgently than you may have thought. Screaming at your partner or kicking the cat is misdirected and pointless. Running away, though, is no better. Better instead to recognise these symptoms of stress before it comes to this. Better physically, better socially and better for your psychological and spiritual health. So try to stop taking out your own tensions on other people. Stop blaming others and stop making excuses for your own less than perfect behaviour. Try not to retire into your shell completely either. These are all unhelpful defence mechanisms which hamper progress and stunt personal growth.

Start by abandoning all negative thoughts, remember that your pessimism is not borne out by the true facts. There are other ways of looking at every situation and there is a good side to most things. Unhelpful thoughts can hinder rather than help you and just because one little thing goes wrong it is not a disaster and it doesn't change everything else. Focus on your strengths rather than your weaknesses, and praise rather than blame yourself. It is so very easy to allow matters to get out of proportion or to attempt to shoulder all the responsibility when problems arise, but resist it. Instead, develop more positive responses that you could substitute for each critical thought so you learn to see each problem in a different, more constructive, light. Practise these positive responses and call on them for each similar situation in the future.

Let go of your stress by becoming a calmer person. Ease up and stop rushing everywhere. Finish one task at a time, wait patiently when you have to without wasting useful energy by tapping your feet, clenching your teeth or biting your nails. Do things more slowly. Do things which show your partner or children that you love them. Understand and control your own anger. Read more, take a soothing bath for twenty minutes and practise a short relaxation routine whenever the chaos and challenges around you become too oppressive. Remember that each new day is a new beginning, a fresh opportunity to start again. No matter how distressing the events of yesterday they belong in the past, and whilst it is easy sometimes to wake up in dread of the new challenges today might bring, the imagined fear is often much worse than the situation or task when you actually come to confront it in reality. The burdens of the day ahead can sometimes seem monstrous, immense, innumerable and unremitting, but you can and you will deal with them. Just keep the issues in perspective. Try to focus on the big picture and establish your real priorities today, then take each small step at a time. Here are my top 50 quick-fix tips for beating stress.

1. Keep count of stressful events in your life.
2. Spend more time on those neglected hobbies.
3. Practise relaxation techniques.
4. Make a long-term life plan.

5. Learn to delegate.

6. Spend more time with family and friends.

7. Allow yourself more time to unwind.

8. Cut back on fatty food.

9. Avoid perfectionism.

10. Establish your priorities.

11. Stay within sensible drinking limits.

12. Put social time for yourself in your appointment diary.

13. Ensure that you are enjoying your job.

14. Do one task at a time and finish it.

15. Hug somebody regularly.

16. Enjoy a walk-break every day.

17. Accept your own faults and weaknesses.

18. Avoid setting unnecessary deadlines.

19. Smile more.

20. Be realistic about your goals and ambitions.

21. Cut your caffeine intake.

22. Accept other people's faults and weaknesses.

23. Speak and walk more slowly.

24. Seek help from others when you need it.

25. Organise your day to day activity more constructively.

26. Buy someone a gift.

27. Practise anger control using a relaxation exercise.

28. Write to a friend.

29. Write down a list of any outstanding jobs to free your mind.

30. Leave your watch off on Sundays.

31. Think positively.

32. Snack on healthy foods, not junk foods.

33. Be more assertive.

34. Eliminate time wasters from your life.
35. Practise mental rehearsals to prepare you for difficult situations.
36. Don't be forced to make on-the-spot decisions.
37. Cut back interruptions and distractions to a minimum.
38. Handle phone calls on your own terms – call back if necessary.
39. Reschedule appointments to coincide with times when you feel at your best.
40. Don't bother getting angry about things you cannot change.
41. Laugh and play more every day.
42. Take regular fun exercise.
43. Cut back or give up smoking.
44. Communicate stress by sharing it with a friend or associate whom you trust.
45. In crisis meetings handle the emotions first, think about the content later.
46. Take a 'nice person' break: when under pressure find someone who lifts your spirits to spend time with.
47. Keep things in perspective: how serious is the situation really?
48. Move on when you have done your best, don't dwell and linger on something when there is nothing more you can do.
49. Practise being a good listener.
50. Finally, praise and encourage others when they have done well.

Complementary Therapies

Interest in alternative medicine and the popularity of complementary therapies is booming. In recent years vastly increasing numbers of people have turned to sources of healing beyond the realms of recognised conventional treatment. Ironically, many family doctors have even learned the art of hypnosis, acupuncture, homeopathy and other techniques, and several of their fraternity even regard themselves as spiritual healers. Other doctors have not gone so far as to incorporate these skills into their own therapeutic repertoire but are happy to employ outside therapists to help in their busy clinics. The regulatory bodies which control the medical profession have also recently adopted a much less stand-offish approach to certain sections of complementary medicine.

The cost of complementary therapy can be substantial but it is nevertheless regarded by many as offering gentler, more natural and safer options than traditional medicine. This attitude may be controversial but the fact that complementary therapies tend to put the patient more in control of their destiny is beyond doubt.

For women going through the menopause, complementary therapies have much to offer. Some conventional doctors will dismiss complementary therapies, but it is still worth pursuing the matter if you feel that is the right course of treatment for you. For women with a variety of physical and psychological symptoms of the change, attitudes vary between very negative or very positive towards it. A complementary healer may appear to listen to what the patient feels about the cause of her own problems and be less likely than a conventionally trained doctor to try to contradict her interpretation. This often makes women feel that the complementary therapist is more on their side. Lifestyle factors are much more likely to be taken into account and a much greater proportion of the advice and treatment given by the therapist is devoted to suggested alternatives to the way patients lead their lives on an everyday basis. Many menopausal women welcome this. Family doctors try as hard as they can to adopt an holistic approach to helping patients, but in view of the sheer number of patients they see on a daily basis, and the level of expectation upon them, they find it hard to achieve. Complementary therapists always regard each patient as a whole entity, seeing individuals as unique and special. This contrasts with the conventional process of categorising patients according to their condition, and allows for different perspectives and more than one single truth. It enables the therapist to respond to people in terms of their body, mind and spirit within the context of their family, their culture and their environment. In addition, an holistic approach could be applied to a wide variety of therapies including drugs and surgery while embracing meditation, diet, massage and manipulation.

A large number of complementary therapies can be applied to the menopause of which, in my experience, the following ten are amongst the most effective and popular as well as being the best researched.

1. Relaxation

Relaxation is a skill that everybody should master. It is a vital element in leading a healthy lifestyle and its benefits are many and varied. Its importance has been recognised for centuries as part of the Eastern philosophies, and nowadays more and more people in the West are beginning to practise relaxation techniques. This includes the conventional medical profession, who are becoming increasingly aware of its advantages to their patients.

Relaxation impinges on part of the nervous system which can be acutely altered at the time of the menopause. It controls our heartbeat, regulates our breathing, controls skin temperature and normalises digestive processes. It brings about sleep and a sense of peace and tranquillity. It is the relaxation response which is the opposite of the stress response, and triggering it can ease muscular tension, reduce blood pressure and cholesterol levels, improve circulation where blood flow to the skin and other organs is restricted, and ease hot flushes and night sweats which can be so troublesome in mid-life. It can also help people suffering from panic attacks and anxiety. It banishes tension from muscles and joints, and together with meditation can ease a troubled mind to bring about spiritual awareness and fulfilment. Mental well-being can be enhanced along with alertness and concentration. Memory and creativity may also receive a boost. Above all, relaxation means that people can become less dependent on artificial sedatives such as tranquillisers, anti-depressants and hypnotic drugs. It provides time out from the turmoil and chaos going on around us, a chance for the human body and spirit to recharge its chronically drained batteries.

There are many varied techniques which you can adapt to help to relax you but whichever you choose it should be practised on a regular basis in order to gain maximum benefit for your psychological and physical health. Frequent use of a relaxation technique will also make it much easier for you to handle episodes of acutely intense stress, the kind of stress which leads to so many unpleasant symptoms.

Prepare for deep muscular relaxation by finding a quiet place where you will not be disturbed by anybody or by the telephone. This place should be warm and quiet. Close the curtains and turn off the light. Now carry out the following steps.

1. Put on some relaxing music. Lie on a comfortable flat surface with a pillow supporting your head and another under your knees if you wish. Close your eyes, settle yourself into the most comfortable position you can find, legs slightly apart and hands loosely by your sides.
2. Now focus on the muscles of your abdomen. Feel the tension unwinding and flowing away. Let the small of your back touch the floor and the muscles go completely limp and loose.
3. Breathe slowly and deeply, let all thoughts leave your mind. Concentrate slowly on the music you are playing and how weightless you feel. Relax and feel at peace.
4. Now focus on the muscles of your arms, let them feel heavy yet weightless. Allow them to hang loosely by your sides and feel the tension flow from your fingertips.
5. Relax and breathe slowly and deeply. Feel all of your body completely relax. Breathe slowly and deeply.
6. Now focus on the muscles in your legs. Let them lie completely unsupported on the floor. Allow them to be heavy, dull, yet weightless. Be completely aware of the lack

of tension in all of your body. Breathe slowly and deeply. Feel calm and relaxed.

7. Now feel how all of your body is completely relaxed. Suspended in weightlessness. Completely relaxed. Breathe slowly and deeply.
8. Allow your breath to leave your lungs completely as you breathe out each time. Allow your chest to collapse and then take a new deep breath.
9. Repeat the process over and over again. Always slowly. Breathe deeply and slowly, relax and savour the sensation. Now you have achieved complete relaxation and are free of all tension. You will feel both relaxed and content.

This deep muscular relaxation technique concentrates on calming the body physically. Women who feel that their menopausal symptoms are mainly psychological may wish to try meditation in addition. Again, a quiet environment and a comfortable position is essential.

1. Kick off your shoes and loosen any tight clothing.
2. Now consciously let go and be aware of the silence around you as well as the gentle ebb and flow of your breathing.
3. Breathe in and out gently through your nose. As you breathe out say a word which is a personal secret word or sound that should have no emotional meaning but which conveys a feeling of peace and serenity. Choose a word similar in imagery to 'sea'. Now as you breathe out say the word 'sea' silently to yourself.
4. Breathe in again, gently repeating the word 'sea' as you exhale. Carry on doing this, concentrating only on your breathing and the repetition of the word 'sea'. Clear your mind totally of all distractions. If you find that your mind wanders or that distracting thoughts start to intrude on your concentration, take yourself back to your breathing and the word 'sea'. Force out those distractions and try not to follow them.

5. Carry on meditating like this for five minutes at a time until you find it easy to clear your mind of all distractions.

With enough practice you will gradually be able to increase your meditation time for up to 20 minutes. If you can find a specific time every day to go through this technique it will more than repay itself in terms of potential benefit, helping you to cope with stressful situations by remaining calm and unfazed. The ideal time to do it is first thing in the morning or last thing at night.

2. Massage

Massage therapy involves the physical application of touch to the soft tissues of the body to promote well-being and health. It is safe, relaxing and gentle, and because it involves a touch between the therapist and the patient it is able to bring them closer together with an emotional and physical bond that is impossible to achieve in any distant or remote way. Some forms of treatment are very gentle and soothing whereas others are powerful, forceful and at times even slightly uncomfortable. Massage can be applied to the body as a whole or it can focus on particular areas such as the head and neck. Massage helps to relax muscles and break down muscular tension and pain. For menopausal women the benefits of massage may be considerable. Not only does it ease painful joints and muscles, but it can reduce emotional tension too. Researchers at Harvard Medical School found that when massage was used in conjunction with pre-operative counselling and advice, patients required less pain relief post-operatively and were discharged from hospital several days earlier than patients who were given the same information without the massage.

In clinical studies massage has been able to lift depression in some patients and improve insomnia and anxiety. It conveys a wonderful feeling of well-being and peace and is a terrific adjunct to a healthy lifestyle which incorporates regular exercise and a healthy diet. There are many different types of massage, probably the one known best in Britain being Swedish massage. Other kinds based on oriental massage, such as Reike and Tuina, are related to spiritual healing through lighter touch. Women using massage to help with their menopause, or even just using it generally, can either employ the services of a professionally trained therapist, or equally well teach themselves massage of a simple kind and then practise it on a partner or another member of the family. The technique is simple enough. All you have to do is follow these simple steps.

1. Use a warm, quiet, dark room where there are no distractions.
2. Remove any watches or jewellery which could scratch the skin.
3. Expose the area to be massaged.
4. Make sure the skin is clear of infection or inflammation and that whatever pain there is is not made worse or does not spread to other areas when pressure is applied.
5. The person being massaged should lie on a firm padded surface.
6. Ideally use an aromatherapy massage oil so your hands can glide smoothly over the skin. A light vegetable oil or talcum powder can be used instead.
7. Pour no more than one teaspoonful of massage oil into the palm of one hand and warm the oil by rubbing your hands together.
8. Begin with circular movements, moulding your hands to the shape of the body and maintaining a constant rhythm.
9. Keep one hand in contact with the skin at all times. If more oil is needed pour a little on to the back of the massaging hand and continue stroking as you use your other hand to transfer the oil on to the recipient's skin.
10. Keep conversation to a minimum during the massage.
11. On small areas use only thumb and fingertips.
12. On large areas use the whole hand and firmer pressure.
13. If massage causes tickling, either increase the pressure or go on to different parts.

14. If muscle tone is being treated the thumbs should exert deep pressure and move in small circles.
15. To relieve tension in muscles around the shoulder or pelvic girdle or thighs, a kneading technique can be used which involves pummelling with the edge of the hand to create a chopping, bouncing effect on the muscles.

Further information can be obtained from the British Massage Therapy Council (see Useful Addresses).

3. Aromatherapy

Possibly the fastest growing of all the complementary therapies, aromatherapy has even moved into NHS hospitals and hospices for the treatment of a whole range of symptoms including sleep disorders, stress and anxiety and pain control. As a soother and calmer, or even sometimes as an invigorator, it has an excellent place in the management of the menopause.

Aromatherapy is thought to stimulate the brain in ways which alter the release of neurotransmitters and hormones such as endorphins which are the body's natural opiates and which give us a lift or a high when we are stimulated by such things as exercise or great joy. Aromatherapy literally means 'treatment using scent'. The therapy exploits the various healing capacities of various plant oils, which may be derived from petals or other parts of the flower, from twigs of trees and from fruit, bark, seeds or grasses. The plant oils consist of tiny droplets in the plant material which are given off in greater concentrations in particular seasons and at certain times of the day or night.

Aromatherapy is designed as a treatment to enhance psychological and physical health, and to promote emotional and somatic well-being. In doing so it is thought to be helpful in avoiding any imbalance in the body's energy systems and in preventing illness and disease. The oils are usually applied by skin massage but can also be used in inhalation therapy in baths, in oil burners, or in the form of cold compresses applied directly to the skin. Aromatherapy is especially helpful for stress-related conditions including anxiety and depression, but is also of benefit when combined with massage for muscular skeletal problems such as muscle aching and rheumatic pain. It is helpful for period problems, fluid retention, digestive disorders and, in particular, problems relating to the menopause. Essential oils particularly recommended include clary sage, cypress, geranium, jasmine, neroli and rose otto. Use oils that are pure and natural as the cheaper ones are not so effective.

4. Herbal medicine

The use of herbs as medicine has been known to all cultures for thousands of years and must be one of the oldest therapies of all. Not only has herbalism been popular in the West but it has also formed an integral part of ancient Chinese medicine and of African and Indian therapies since the beginning of time. Herbal preparations derived from flowers, roots, barks, seeds and nuts consist of a number of different chemical components that are known to have curative properties in humans. The remedies themselves come in many shapes and forms. They can be taken orally or rubbed on the skin, and they come as tinctures, decoctions, infusions, tablets, capsules, compresses, poultices and herbal baths. Each is made up differently.

Although it is possible to buy an over-the-counter herbal remedy, this goes against the grain to some extent because herbal therapists believe that treatment should be tailored to the individual and should not be dispensed empirically with a particular illness in mind. Many people require guidance, at least to begin with, in selecting the correct treatment, and are therefore happy to book an appointment with a trained herbalist. Contact the London School of Aromatherapy (see Useful Addresses) for further information. Long experience relating to women troubled by symptoms of the menopause highlights the following herbal remedies as being particularly worthy of attention. They are each worth trying in turn, and they include:

Sage (Salvia officianalis). Sage can be useful in the treatment of night sweats and hot flushes, particularly the ones that produce profuse perspiration, as it is a plant with an affinity for drying out that which is too wet. It should be avoided by women who are experiencing vaginal dryness or a dry mouth. It can be used either as dried sage burned in a room or as an infusion (one teaspoon of dried leaves in a cup of hot water is left to sit for ten minutes, then one tablespoon of the cooled mixture can be taken one to eight times a day). Alternatively, you can use 10 to 25 drops of tincture of sage every day. Sage may also be used in cooking, sprinkled over steamed or wok-fried vegetables and salads, in cooked grains, soups and casseroles. Sage is thought to be able to calm anxiety, banish depression and balance mood. It is good for helping to fight infections, improve digestion, relieve heavy periods, ease inflammation and relieve headaches.

Alfalfa. Alfalfa is rich in isoflavones, coumarins and sterols and has an action similar to the other phytoestrogens. Alfalfa also yields ten times more mineral value than average grains. It is helpful in reducing cholesterol levels, preventing anaemia and promoting strong and healthy bones and teeth. It may be drunk as a tea, taken as a liquid extract or even as a green drink (fresh alfalfa is passed through a blender after which the juice is then drunk in doses of about a wine-glassful). Taken regularly it is thought to dispose towards mental and physical well-being.

Vervain. This herb was sacred to the Greeks and Druids and is thought to be particularly helpful for emotional symptoms. It is antispasmodic, used for the relief of tension and stress. It is therefore particularly good for the psychological consequences of the menopause and has been used for post-operative depression, agoraphobia and other social phobias, and general nervous exhaustion.

Panax Ginseng. Some believe this herb to be the most effective of all herbs for the relief of very severe and debilitating symptoms of the menopause. It is widely cultivated in China, Korea, Japan and Russia, and has been highly thought of for centuries in view of its rejuvenating properties, its ability to protect against illness, to enhance the body's ability to handle stress, and even to prolong life expectancy. Vitamin E seems to enhance its action whereas high doses of vitamin C can reduce it. Its wild root is the most effective form and it can be chewed or a tincture may be made from it. For menopausal women panax ginseng is especially useful as it is helpful in regulating hormones and preventing menstrual flooding. It also boosts energy levels and improves a woman's ability to handle stress.

Dong Quai – Angelica Sinensis. A sister to ginseng and containing less than a quarter of a per cent of the amount of oestrogen found in pharmaceutical HRT drugs, dong quai is famous amongst herbalists for quickly being able to reduce hot flushes and night sweats. It may also calm menopausal anxiety, boost metabolism, protect the circulation and heart, and ease insomnia, anxiety and depression. Acting more quickly than ginseng, which takes up to eight weeks to provide its full benefit, dong quai is often prescribed for a fortnight followed by ginseng for the next fortnight, and so on. Dong quai can be chewed in the dried root form three times a day, or taken as an infusion or fresh fruit tincture. Whilst easing hot flushes and moistening a dry vagina, it is best avoided in women who have abdominal bloating, menstrual flooding or breast tenderness. One randomised clinical trial of dong quai found it to be no more effective than placebo.

Chaste Tree or Vitex Agnus Castus. Also known as Monk's Pepper, this herb has been claimed by some herbalists to stimulate sex drive in women and energise her whole system whilst controlling emotional mood swings. It can be taken as an infusion, in powdered form, in capsules or as a tincture. It is thought to be particularly effective in eliminating hot flushes, regulating periods and easing cramps, moistening the vagina, strengthening bones, easing constipation and eliminating depression.

Black Cohosh, otherwise known as Cimicifuga Racemosa. Also called black snake root or Sheng Ma in Chinese herbal medicine, this plant has been used for hundreds of years by native Americans to treat conditions of the female reproductive system and also of the menopause. It can be taken as a decoction or as a tincture, and is particularly good for calming hot flushes, easing generalised aches and pains and heightening energy whilst calming nerves. It should be avoided in pregnancy and in women suffering from heavy menstrual bleeding.

Motherwort or Leonurus Cardiaca. This herb, otherwise known as Yim U Cao or Lion's tail in Chinese medicine, is used to calm the nerves, reduce hot flushes, promote good sound refreshing sleep and to tone up the womb and vagina. It is thought to have natural diuretic properties too, and can be taken as an infusion, as a tincture or as a herbal vinegar. As motherwort can aggravate menstrual flooding, however, it should be avoided by women with heavy periods.

Golden Seal – Hydrastis Canadensis. A popular cure-all with the Cherokee Indians, golden seal is now used widely in the West to regulate digestion and liver disorders, to fight infections and to ease menstrual cramps. It is sometimes used as a douche in the treatment of vaginal infections and can also ease skin disorders and haemorrhoids. It can be taken in powdered root form, in capsules or by infusion.

Wild Yam – Dioscorea Villosa. Wild yam, as the whole plant, provides the raw materials which enable the body to make hormones and has much to offer women who are peri-menopausal. Some doctors believe that the menopause, rather than being a condition of oestrogen deficiency, is more a condition brought about by reduced progesterone levels relative to the amount of oestrogen, and thus they regard it as a condition of relative oestrogen dominance. Since wild yam may boost the production of natural progesterone, it is prescribed to moisten the vagina, ease itching and burning in that area, and to prevent emotional ups and downs in the post-menopausal period. The views of American Dr John Lee, its prime advocate, remain controversial but he believes it can reverse osteoporosis and have a beneficial effect on many of the physical and psychological symptoms of the menopause. As it can do little harm you may wish to try it; many have done with good therapeutic results anecdotally.

5. Bach flower remedies

Dr Edward Bach gave up his thriving conventional medical practice in Harley Street in 1930 to pursue a unique interest. He had often escaped the confines of London to go for long walks in the countryside and was struck by how walking through woods and fields in the fresh air could relax and revitalise him. He was drawn especially to particular flowers and began to experiment with the effect of dew taken from those he came across. Starting with an initial 12 remedies, he added more by soaking flower petals in spring water, and eventually developed 38 flower remedies for the benefit of every possible personality, state of mind and emotional state. Like homeopathic medicines, Bach flower remedies contain no detectable or recognisable ingredients from the original plant or flower. Flower therapists explain that each remedy contains merely the imprint of the flower from which it was derived and that the energy contained within the remedy acts as a catalyst to trigger the body's innate healing powers. Although no randomised clinical trials have substantiated the therapeutic claims of these remedies, plenty of anecdotal evidence from many a satisfied customer suggests that they do have an important part to play in treatment. Where the menopause has been complicated by psychological difficulties and emotional sources of stress, including anxiety, depression, loneliness, grief and bereavement, trying them can certainly cause no harm. One of the most well-known examples is Rescue Remedy which is a mixture of several different ingredients, namely star of Bethlehem, impatiens, cherry, plum, clematis and rock rose. It is designed for people in emotional crises, for patients who feel shocked, out of control, mentally numb or in turmoil and panic. Many menopausal and post-menopausal women swear by it.

6. Chiropractic and osteopathy

Both of these treatments involve physical manipulation of the body's bones, ligaments, joints and muscles in order to diagnose problems, alleviate pain, enhance mobility and improve general health. Based on the belief that structure governs function, the manipulative techniques are employed not just to influence the parts of the muscular skeletal system being re-aligned and physically altered, but to improve function in peripheral and distant organs as well.

Many people are confused as to the subtle differences between osteopathy and chiropractic treatment, but in fact they are fairly clear. Osteopaths work on all areas of the body whereas chiropractors tend to concentrate on the spine. Osteopaths rarely use x-rays whereas chiropractors often call upon them. Osteopaths use soft tissue techniques, such as muscle massage, to a greater degree than chiropractors. Remember that manipulative therapy is also performed by physiotherapists whose work is available free of charge on the NHS. For menopausal women with general aches and pains, fibrositis, muscle stiffness, arthritis or tension headaches, these manipulative techniques can provide considerable and often very dramatic relief without recourse to more powerful drugs. At a time in a woman's life when she should be very conscious of her bones and her skeleton, osteopathy and chiropractic are treatments well worth considering. See Useful Addresses for details of the headquarters of the national organisations.

7. Alexander technique

The Alexander Technique is more a form of education than a therapy and consists of a combination of verbal instructions and postural guidance. The idea is to teach the pupil to give up bad habits, such as slumping in the chair, slouching on a sofa, sitting round-shouldered at a desk, and walking with the head bowed or slanting to one side. It is designed to restore in people who have chronically adopted these bad habits the ability to move with the graceful ease of a child, and to teach them how to conduct themselves with enhanced balance and poise. Teachers of the Alexander Technique blame our modern working methods for many of our problems, and certainly our stressful lifestyles and sedentary occupations leave a lot to be desired.

Pupils who have successfully used the Alexander Technique are generally very enthusiastic about its benefits. Having been taught its methods they say they have been rendered free of tension, they feel lighter on their feet and they feel taller and more elegant in the way they move. It is used for treating chronic fatigue and tiredness, breathing disorders, muscular skeletal aches and pains, stress-related conditions such as insomnia and palpitations, and also to boost self-confidence and self-esteem.

8. Reflexology

Reflexology is a therapy which involves the application of pressure to focal points on the feet or hands to encourage the body to heal from within. The various forms of foot massage have been used in India, China and Egypt for over 5,000 years and were also popular amongst the native American Indians and African tribes people. Whether or not energy within the body can really be rebalanced or stimulated from distant parts by applying pressure to the foot as is claimed, there is no doubt that many people benefit from the soothing and calming effect of foot massage. Reflexology is carried out with a view to boosting energy levels and enhancing emotional and spiritual well-being. It can ease tension headaches, migraines, high blood pressure, irritable bowel syndrome, skin disorders such as psoriasis and eczema, and may be useful too in treating back pain and menstrual irregularities.

9. Yoga

Yoga is a gentle discipline from which even the disabled, the arthritic, the elderly and the terminally ill can draw benefit. It is an exercise system which enhances the psyche as well as the soma, and is a great way of promoting union between the mind and the body. The postures adopted in yoga can increase suppleness and strength, but the philosophy behind it and the relaxation it engenders is designed to alleviate stress and to counter negative emotions which can be commonplace at the time of the menopause. Yoga can be highly beneficial in treating both physical and psychological symptoms, in particular anxiety, tension, depression, and all those stress-related conditions like high blood pressure, indigestion, insomnia, palpitations, tremor, poor concentration and lack of confidence.

10. Acupuncture

Acupuncture forms a large part of traditional Chinese medicine and essentially involves inserting extremely fine needles into the skin at specific locations known as acupoints, which can be used to alter the balance of energy throughout the body. It can be both an holistic treatment, designed to alter the body's own natural healing energy and bring about well-being, good health and long life from within; or it can be used more specifically as in Western or scientific acupuncture, to treat particular complaints such as pain, arthritis or insomnia. So effective has it proved that it is now being widely adopted in most NHS hospitals to relieve a large number of medical complaints. Conventionally trained users of acupuncture believe it works within the nervous system by releasing substances which are naturally produced opiate pain killers, and which have a powerful effect on the sensation of pain. These are the same endorphins or happy hormones that are enhanced after regular exercise or excitement, and their presence may be the reason why people do not feel the pain of even a severe injury when it is incurred in the heat of battle, during sudden trauma or on the playing field. Acupuncture is employed for an enormous range of emotional, physical and psychological problems including the menopause, menstrual problems, high blood pressure, insomnia, depression, stress and anxiety, irritable bowel syndrome, and a host of other far-ranging conditions.

The Holistic Approach

Complementary therapies lend themselves ideally to the complex web of physical, psychological and cultural consequences of the menopause. Often you may well be able to cope with the physical inconvenience brought about by falling oestrogen levels, but there remains a need to make sense of the changes which you are experiencing and a desire to put them into perspective. Not all women will require medication, as such, for their problems, and the holistic approach to the menopause offered by many complementary practitioners can satisfy many of the psychological doubts and social worries which can surface at this time.

Provided they find a reputable therapist who is experienced, well qualified, registered with one of the recognised national organisations, and who provides some kind of professional indemnity for their clients, even the most conventionally orientated of menopausal women can be surprisingly impressed by what complementary therapists have to offer.

PART FOUR

CHAPTER 13

HORMONE REPLACEMENT THERAPY –
THE BENEFITS

HRT is something which replaces the hormones that a woman's body stops producing after the menopause. Because it alleviates many of the uncomfortable and inconvenient symptoms of a moderate or severe menopause it is also considered as a form of therapy.

The Origins of HRT

The origins of HRT derive from the culmination of a lifetime's work by Dr Robert A. Wilson. Dr Wilson was English. He grew up in the final years of the nineteenth century in Lancashire. He recalled with sadness how much the health of his mother and other women at that time had declined in their peri-menopausal and post-menopausal years, and having moved to the USA it took him more than 40 years of work and investigation to become established as the originator of hormone replacement therapy.

In the 1920s the hormone oestrogen was identified and by the late 1930s synthetic oestrogen was being made. Experimental work during the 1940s led to the clinical introduction of oestrogens in the USA in the 1950s, and then Britain and other countries followed just a few years later. Dr Wilson clarified the various potential benefits of successful long-term usage of this therapy, most of which has been confirmed by further studies in more recent years.

Ever since the 1940s doctors have been prescribing HRT to women whose ovaries no longer produce normal amounts of oestrogen. Although the oestrogens are given in doses equivalent to the average level produced during the normal menstrual cycle, most forms of HRT provide a fixed dose, which does not exactly recreate the normal premenopausal fluctuations. However, the steady levels of oestrogen provided by HRT may in fact be an advantage, as mood changes, headaches and other symptoms are often related to the ups and downs of premenopausal hormone changes anyway.

Dr Wilson's early work resulted in a form of therapy which was not merely capable of eliminating hot flushes, night sweats and other common menopausal symptoms, but which could also prevent or delay the brittling of bones, heart disease, muscle deterioration, digestive disorders, vaginal dryness and shrinkage, genital irritation and cystitis, pain in joints and even wrinkles in the skin. Dr Wilson himself said, 'HRT is a proven, effective means of restoring the normal balance of [a woman's] bodily and psychic functions throughout her prolonged life.' But even he fully appreciated that HRT would not be suitable for everyone, and that doctors should always fully evaluate a woman's medical history before prescribing it.

Joan Jenkins, the founder of the Women's Health Concern Movement in 1972, remains a great admirer of Dr Wilson's work, and still takes HRT herself as she has done for 28 years or more. She says, 'I have been privileged to take advantage of this tremendous step forward in twentieth-century women's health care . . . like millions of others in my age group I have benefited enormously from prolonged therapy.'

But whilst HRT attracted its devoted advocates, it also attracted its critics. Feminists, for example, and ardent supporters of natural or complementary therapy voiced doubts about whether the menopause should be medicalised at all. They saw it, and still do, as an entirely natural event in a woman's life, which has its own spiritual and evolutionary meaning, and which can be managed by non-pharmacological means. Such sceptics question the idea of oestrogen deficiency and regard HRT purely as a money-spinning proposition designed by a greedy and commercially motivated pharmaceutical industry.

More recently HRT has been described as 'the elixir of eternal youth' and 'the best thing since sliced bread' by thousands of women who, after suffering from severe menopausal symptoms for years, took on a new lease of life as a result of feeling so much younger and fitter again. It was in the light of such clinical improvement in increasing numbers of women, and in the wake of the publication of Dr Wilson's book *Feminine Forever* in 1966, that interest in the treatment of menopausal symptoms continued apace after the 1950s. Since then HRT has remained the cornerstone for treatment of menopausal symptoms and we have established a large body of clinical trial data to support its efficacy in alleviating immediate symptoms and reducing the prevalence of the long-term consequences of the menopause, such as osteoporosis and cardiovascular disease. So whilst the appropriate use of phytoestrogens, certain food supplements, vitamins, minerals and some herbal mixtures can be helpful, and whilst complementary therapies like acupuncture and osteopathy also have their place, the vast majority of scientific opinion agrees that there is still no substitute for HRT to eliminate menopausal symptoms and to protect against the hazards of known oestrogen deficiency.

Why is HRT Prescribed?

For those women suffering from troublesome or inconvenient symptoms of the menopause which significantly affect their quality of life, HRT has much to offer. Hot flushes and night sweats can seriously affect any woman's life and become socially disabling. While many women only suffer mild symptoms and can get by with no treatment or 'complementary' treatment, other women find the relief from symptoms afforded by HRT a god send. When used appropriately, it is certainly the wonder drug many claim it to be.

In my own surgery I have encountered many women who have finally come to see me to talk about how desperate they feel after years of poor health and misery caused by the menopause. I would like to think of myself as a caring and approachable family doctor, yet it might still take great courage and determination for such patients to open up about their feelings and lack of well-being. Some feel guilty about wasting a doctor's time, and many were brought up to believe that the menopause was simply something they got on with and never complained about. It is a woman's lot in life that had to be endured. It is something you didn't moan to the doctor about. It is also embarrassing, somehow, an admission of an inability to cope, and it was stigmatised. Well-publicised feminists and certain minority groups have also loudly denounced women for not accepting the menopause as 'natural' and have even made some women feel even more guilty about seeking medical help.

But the truth is that HRT can revolutionise the life of a woman plagued by serious symptoms of the menopause, and in my own experience as a GP I have found it to be one of the most dramatic therapies available to people in the whole field of modern therapeutics. Just as thyroxine hormone can drastically change the health of a person with an underactive thyroid, or corticosteroids can revive a person with underactive adrenal glands, so HRT can provide a new lease of life to a woman whose ovarian function has waned after the menopause.

The Far-Reaching Benefits of HRT

HRT was once thought to help only certain symptoms of the menopause, notably hot flushes, night sweats, irregular periods and vaginal dryness. These problems, which are demonstrably caused by oestrogen deficiency, respond dramatically to HRT, but increasingly more and more recent research into the uses of HRT has revealed improvements in other physical symptoms, including urinary problems, skin changes, loss of libido, general aches and pains, fatigue, muscle weakness, headaches, IBS and constipation. Even the physiological symptoms, which many consider to be bound up with factors related to age, social role or depression, have now been shown by new scientific endeavours to be responsive to treatment with HRT. In other words, studies have demonstrated a clear mechanism of action as to how and why HRT might work in these various clinical situations. The bottom line is that for almost every single symptom that a woman might experience during the menopause, HRT provides a useful and effective solution.

Further details about the efficacy of HRT for short-term menopausal symptoms can be found below, including the latest fascinating research that HRT really does help keep women looking younger and more shapely. HRT is also prescribed, probably increasingly, for control of long-term complications of the menopause, notably for the prevention of osteoporosis and heart disease. Since coronary heart disease is the single greatest killer of post-menopausal women, any medication offering significant protection against such a condition must be worthy of serious consideration. For women at increased risk because of the presence of a number of contributory factors, such as heavy smoking, diabetes and a strong family history, the pros of HRT can be regarded as being of even greater benefit.

HRT is the gold standard treatment for the prevention and treatment of brittle bone disease too, a condition which will otherwise bring about an osteoporotic fracture in one in three women over the age of 50.

These are the reasons why HRT is prescribed, and each year more and more women are finding out about it and making the decision to prosper from its benefits. It is estimated that at the start of this millennium, one in four women aged between 40 and 64 are taking HRT. Interestingly, the proportion is already higher than this among menopausal women doctors, with two out of five of them currently using HRT, that is twice as many as women generally. Clearly, their broader knowledge and clearer understanding of the benefits versus the risks of HRT accounts for the difference.

The Hormones Involved

The two main ingredients of HRT preparations are oestrogen and progestogen. Some women may be offered testosterone as well but only in very occasional circumstances, as we shall see later. The female body naturally produces three main types of oestrogen, namely 17 beta oestradiol, oestrone and oestriol, and one type of progesterone. The levels of all of these hormones naturally diminish at the time of the menopause and because hormone deficiency brings about the symptoms of the menopause, HRT is designed to counteract the effect of this.

Unfortunately, replacing hormones is not always straightforward. It is not quite as simple as merely providing them in tablet form for women to take orally, because the powerful acids and enzymes in the stomach would destroy their molecular structure and render them useless within the body. To be effective, any relevant hormonal ingredients have to be able to pass through the wall of the intestine and into the bloodstream. They have to pass through the barrier of the gut wall and reach the bloodstream in a biologically active form that can have a measurable effect within the body.

HRT and Your Liver

Furthermore, any ingredients must be able to survive transportation to the liver and metabolism within it, as the main job of the liver is to break down and excrete various substances including steroids and hormones. Any HRT that is going to be effective must endure this 'first pass' through the liver in order to reach the main circulation for transportation around the body and to arrive at the sites where its effect is intended. Because of this, HRT in tablet form is usually of a relatively high dosage in order to overcome the fact that the liver will effectively destroy a high proportion of it very early on. The proportion of hormone remaining will then circulate around the body and, depending on its molecular characteristics and its similarity to the hormones naturally found in the body, it may or may not interact with various hormone receptor sites and trigger hormone-like effects. See Figure 20.

HRT and Hormone Receptor sites

The hormones used in HRT may not be identical to the natural hormone produced within the body, but if they clearly resemble

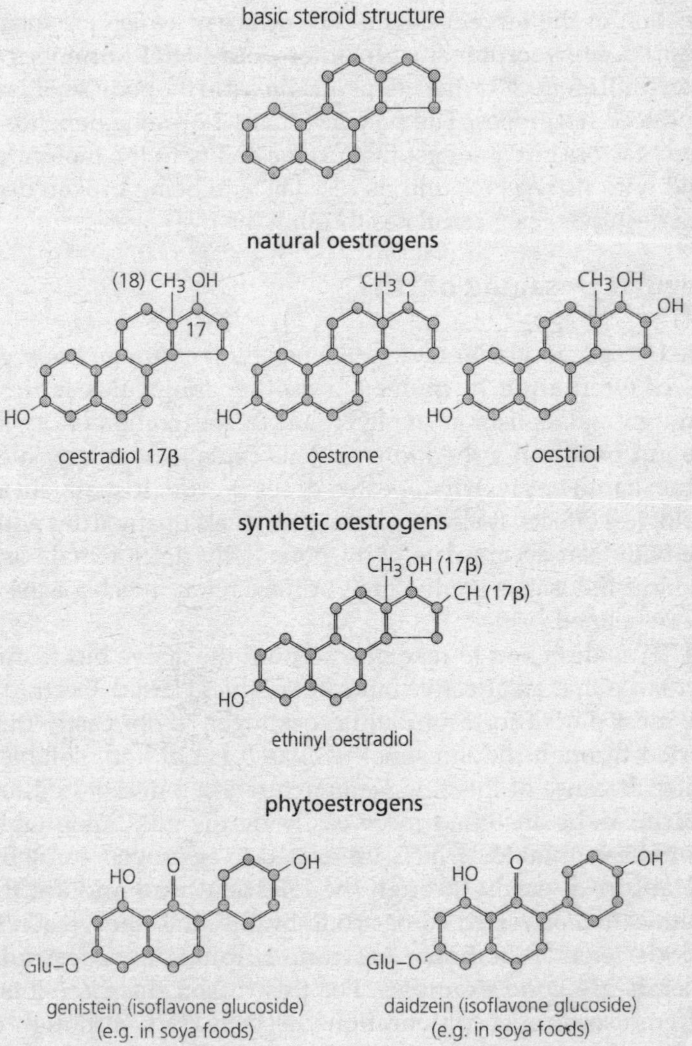

basic steroid structure

natural oestrogens

(18) CH_3 OH CH_3 O CH_3 OH

17   OH

HO   HO   HO

oestradiol 17β   oestrone   oestriol

synthetic oestrogens

CH_3 OH (17β)

CH (17β)

HO

ethinyl oestradiol

phytoestrogens

HO   O   OH   HO   O   OH

Glu–O   Glu–O

genistein (isoflavone glucoside)   daidzein (isoflavone glucoside)
(e.g. in soya foods)   (e.g. in soya foods)

Figure 20

it, they can still fit into the hormone's receptor site like a hand fits in a glove, and in their own right promote changes in the function of the target cells on the surface of which are located these specific receptor sites. In other words, HRT hormones can exert similar effects on the uterus and breast to the body's naturally produced hormones. The potency of any hormone depends on many factors but amongst them is the ability of the molecule to bind with its receptor and its resistance to being broken down and destroyed as it circulates through the liver again.

Regular Dosaging of HRT

The two predominant methods whereby the human body gets rid of circulating hormones and other molecules is firstly through metabolism in the liver and then excretion either into the gut or through the kidneys. This explains why any medication has to be given in repeated doses in order to maintain any biological effects. It also explains why levels of any drug within the body can accumulate, with potentially detrimental consequences if dosages are too high or if excretory mechanisms are overwhelmed.

HRT is designed to take into account the above biochemical factors so that an effective but safe product is used. Oestradiol, the most potent form of natural oestrogen is not easily transported through the intestinal wall as it is not very soluble in water. Because of this it is manufactured in a micronised form which can be absorbed more easily by the gut. Some tablets provide compounds which are related to oestrogen, but which are absorbed easily through the intestinal wall and are then chemically converted to oestrone by the time they reach the bloodstream. Piperazine oestrone sulphate and oestradiol valerate are good examples. For this reason there are lots of different oestrogen preparations used in HRT, although the main active ingredient circulating in the blood is essentially the same.

Progesterone

What about progesterone? Can this hormone be taken orally? The answer is simple: no. The little that is absorbed through the intestine is very rapidly destroyed and has no chance to exert any influence on progesterone receptors leading to progesterone-like effects. For this reason, synthetic forms of progesterone, known as progestogens, are used in HRT; they are biochemically modified versions of the parent molecule and do not have such a rapid metabolism, allowing them to work effectively on progesterone receptors and exert the desirable effect.

Since the various hormones used in HRT possess different biochemical properties, sometimes a more 'natural' (less biochemically modified) hormone can be employed if the HRT is given in a different way. For example, some hormones like oestradiol can be dissolved in alcohol to enable them to be well absorbed through the skin or through the vaginal lining. This is often used in patches, gels and also in subcutaneous implants, in vaginal creams, rings and pessaries. Of course, these non-tablet forms of HRT cannot be applied to all hormones as each is unique and different. One of the advantages they possess is that because they are not absorbed via the digestive system the hormones they contain avoid that destructive 'first pass' through the liver, so the dosages used may be smaller and any potential side effects therefore reduced. The blood levels attained, however, are more or less equivalent. Although natural progesterone is ineffective when given orally and has only a very transient effect when injected, it may still be used and is available in the form of rectal suppositories and vaginal gels.

Many women will have heard about so-called natural progesterone cream such as Progest, derived from wild yam extract, but very little data exists on its physiological effects and it remains particularly controversial. These products are currently 'unlicensed' and there are no randomised clinical trials which show any clear benefits. Initial research suggests that it may have a measurable beneficial effect on controlling hot flushes and night sweats (the predominant vasomotor symptoms of the menopause), but despite circulating literature there is no current evidence that it can prevent osteoporotic bone loss or any of the other long-term complications of the menopause.

Understanding how the various hormones used in HRT work enables doctors to monitor their effects. Blood levels of oestradiol, for example, can be accurately measured in women who have had oestrogen implants (perhaps after a hysterectomy with removal of both ovaries) to see whether the implant needs renewing several months later. If the hormones in a different type of HRT are converted into oestrone in the bloodstream, however, measuring oestradiol will signify very little. In the past it was often commonplace for a woman to be prescribed HRT without any blood test being performed to accurately confirm the menopause nor to monitor the effects of treatment. These days, however, it is much more likely that a scientific approach to HRT, as well as a more compassionate one, will be adopted.

Testosterone HRT

Testosterone has been considered by many doctors to be important in the maintenance of libido in post-menopausal women. In women who have had a surgical menopause, in particular with removal of the ovaries, testosterone levels have been shown to fall by 50 per cent, whereas the usual fall after a natural menopause is only in the region of 20 per cent, because the ovaries still continue to produce small quantities of this hormone thereafter. Women can still report a lack of sex drive after surgery despite being treated with oestrogen-only HRT to prevent vaginal dryness and physical symptoms that might contribute to avoidance of sexual contact, but testosterone certainly seems from many trials to alleviate the problem. Many independent workers in the field of psycho-sexual medicine appear to endorse this view, not only for women who have undergone a surgical menopause but in other women too. There remain doubts about exactly how useful testosterone HRT may be and about the risks of certain unwanted side effects, but medication is available in both oral and injectable form, and may be used either in conjunction with or independently from other forms of HRT.

Is HRT 'Natural'?

If, by the word 'natural', we mean something that would happen 'in the wild' without man's intervention then clearly HRT is not natural. But then nor is treatment for an underactive thyroid, for Parkinson's Disease, for pre-menstrual syndrome, or even as a means of providing contraception for that matter. No medical therapy is 'natural'. That fact alone does not make it bad or undesirable. Equally, there are many events which occur in nature which are deplorable, and many natural substances which are far from therapeutic and which sometimes can be positively dangerous.

On the other hand, if by 'natural' we mean, for example, that a hormone is produced only by the human body then obviously some forms of HRT are natural and others are not. Even that definition may be complicated by the fact that many forms of HRT deliver naturally occurring hormones into the bloodstream, but they start off as compounds which are only related to natural oestrogen and begin life as a synthetically produced analogue of the real thing. Whether this kind of HRT is natural or not is a moot point. From a physiological point of view it most probably is.

Premarin – a More 'Natural' Form of HRT

What about another commonly prescribed type of HRT containing 'natural' conjugated oestrogens? How natural are they? These, in fact, are derived from pregnant mares' urine and as such are equine oestrogens coming from a 'natural' source. The source actually provides this type of HRT with its brand name: Premarin from *pregnant mares' urine*. This form of HRT contains a unique complex of 10 biologically active compounds in which just over 50 per cent of the mixture is made up of oestrone sulphate and the rest of equine equilin sulphate. The latter is converted to equilin in the human body, and because it is structurally very similar to human oestrogen and has an equivalent capacity to bring about hormonal effects on the target receptors, it is considered by doctors to be 'natural'. In fact it is not identical to human oestrogen but very similar in structure and effects. Since all other oestrogens are, to varying degrees, manufactured synthetically from chemicals and contain only one, two or three oestrogens (piperazine oestrone sulphate, 17 beta oestrone and oestradiol valerate) this is the nearest HRT can possibly get to being absolutely natural.

Some women may have reservations about horses being farmed for the purpose of providing HRT. There are always alternatives of course, but in fact horses are used in the production of natural conjugated oestrogens because mares are one of the few mammals which produce high levels of oestrogens during pregnancy that are very similar to those produced by women. Several seem to be unique to pregnant mares, making them the only suitable source of natural conjugated oestrogen.

To reassure women who may have been offered this kind of HRT, and who may have ethical concerns, some information about collection techniques may be helpful. The major pharmaceutical companies which produce this form of HRT contract independent family-run horse ranches in Canada and North America, staffed and owned by experienced horse farmers, many of whom have been breeding horses for generations to produce pregnant mares' urine. The farmers work under strict controls and comply with the Government's code of practice for animal care, developed in co-operation with veterinarians, agricultural nutritionists and others. There is a continuous improvement programme, and an Equine Advisory Board has been set up to advise in all areas of animal husbandry and welfare including nutrition, exercise, physiology and veterinary care. The board members are recognised equine experts and faculty experts at veterinary and agricultural universities. This insures that the mares are well cared for. No other type of livestock farming has as many checks on the standards of animal care and welfare, with inspectors visiting all farms at least once a month.

The urine is collected through a rubber pouch fitted to the mare. The pouch allows freedom of movement without any irritation. The urine is collected only over a relatively short period during pregnancy when oestrogen levels are high. When each mare delivers her foal the two of them are kept together, and over the normal period of a few months the foal is weaned and raised for a number of different purposes such as showing, riding work and breeding.

In terms of HRT production, the component oestrogen in the mares' urine has to be blended and refined, a complex process involving many stages. Stringent testing takes place at each one to ensure the purity of the finished product. Certainly no urine remains in the end product. Finally, after blending, the natural conjugated oestrogens are converted to a fine powder which is then made into tablets and coated.

Even having read this, there may be some women who feel they would prefer to rely on forms of HRT in which the oestrogens come from other natural sources such as cacti or soya bean. In fact these natural oestrogens have also been synthesised in a laboratory, just as some forms of natural progesterone have, although some people still regard them as natural because they have been processed to become identical to those hormones manufactured within the human body itself. Even the phyto-estrogens in plants which we grow and eat cannot be regarded as purely natural, as in molecular terms they are less similar than the horse oestrogen equilin to hormones produced in the body. Looking at the different molecular structures in Figure 20 it can be seen that these oestrogens do not even have the typical steroid rings of other hormones.

Synthetic Oestrogens

So much for natural oestrogens, what about the synthetic forms of oestrogen? These chemically manufactured hormones include ethinyl-oestradiol, mestranol and dienoestrol, which are not converted into hormones identical to those found within the body. These synthetic hormones have structural differences to natural oestradiol, which means that when taken orally, in tablet form, they are metabolised by the liver more slowly and their effects in the body are therefore magnified. So potent are these synthetic hormones that even in small doses they are capable of preventing pregnancy, unlike other forms of HRT which rely on natural oestrogens and do not have the capacity to act as a contraceptive.

Most types of HRT contain the so-called natural oestrogens described above rather than the stronger synthetic ones whereas, by contrast, synthetic forms of *progesterone* are almost always used in conventional HRT. Since there are clearly a number of choices, some women may ask themselves whether it is more natural to take HRT in some other form than in the form of tablets. Sometimes oestradiol skin patches and implants may be considered more natural as the method of absorption means that the hormones trickle into the body slowly, which is more physiological, mirroring what actually happens in the woman's own body. This may be considered better than the peaks and troughs of hormone blood levels which are achieved after ingestion of a tablet. Certainly one of the benefits of HRT patches is that the liver will not encounter a sudden rush of hormone all at one time, and that a better ratio of oestradiol and oestrone is achieved in the bloodstream. But again this definition of natural is debatable. At the end of the day, suffice it to say that there are many options available to women considering HRT, some of which fit into their way of thinking more comfortably than others. Taking insulin as a diabetic, or thyroxine when there is thyroid deficiency, is not entirely natural, and both therapeutic hormones are created synthetically. Without them, however, the quality and quantity of life would be significantly curtailed.

How Does HRT Differ to the Oral Contraceptive Pill?

Many of the worries associated with HRT have come about because women confuse it with the mode of action of the oral contraceptive pill. In fact the hormones used in each are entirely different. The oral contraceptive pill contains high doses of synthetic oestrogens which can be up to eight times more potent than the natural oestrogens used in HRT. Higher doses are needed in the oral contraceptive pill to prevent the ovaries releasing an egg each month at ovulation, therefore bringing about a contraceptive effect. These synthetic oestrogens have the disadvantage of making the blood more sticky which can increase the risk of blood clots in veins, which in turn can sometimes lead to heart attacks and strokes.

HRT, in contrast, has minimal effects on blood clotting and the doses used are equivalent to the amounts produced naturally by the body in the normal menstrual cycle. In fact the natural oestrogens used in HRT reduce the risk of clots in arteries so heart attacks and strokes are actually less likely to occur. The chances of a clot in the veins of a woman taking HRT are the same as those a woman would run during her reproductive years, although the risk is still greater than it would be for a post-menopausal woman who is *not* using HRT. For these reasons, women who were unable to take the oral contraceptive pill before the menopause can often safely take HRT after it. The differences between the oral contraceptive pill and HRT are summarised in Figure 21.

Figure 21

**Differences between the oral contraceptive pill
and oestrogen replacement**

Oral contraceptive pill	Oestrogen replacement (HRT)
Contains synthetic oestrogens	Usually contains natural oestrogens
Contains high doses of oestrogens	Contains low doses of oestrogens
Increases the risk of blood clots and thromboses	Minimal effects on blood clotting

How Do We Know HRT Works?

Orthodox medical practice may have been guilty in recent years for not providing an holistic approach towards people and their medical conditions, but at least it has established a sound and often irrefutable scientific foundation to support and justify its methods and practices. Ever since the 1940s, randomised medical trials have been employed to demonstrate scientifically and accurately whether any new drug, treatment or surgical intervention of any kind is effective, safe and superior to or at least as good as any existing therapies. These trials also reveal any side effect or adverse reaction caused by the treatment that might not have been suspected from experimentation on animals. Randomised clinical trials are very carefully set up expressly to eliminate any misleading results. Personal bias and a placebo effect (where a person's expectations of a treatment alter the way the person perceives the effect) must be ruled out if the trial is to be of any true value, and the randomised trial effectively achieves just that. Certainly no better or more reliable method of evaluation has ever been described. By the time the results have also been subjected to rigorous and repeated statistical analysis, scientists are generally prepared to accept that the treatment really does work because the results and observations witnessed are repeatable and verifiable by other researchers. In other words, the constancy and reliability of the results can be re-tested and re-proved. Not only is the randomised clinical trial reliable, it has also been invaluable for detecting which treatments are best for patients. It has shown the medical profession how best to treat those with breast cancer or leukaemia, for example, whether one drug is better than another and whether symptoms of a disease are a side effect of the treatment or a complication of the disease itself.

There are different types of randomised clinical trials: prospective ones which follow people into the future, and retrospective ones which depend on individuals within the trial recalling their symptoms and how they felt in the past. There are 'blind' trials, which refers to the fact that the doctors handing out the treatments do not know themselves which are the active treatments and which are the dummy treatments, and the set up of such studies is closely administered and monitored by authoritative ethical committees.

The bigger the trial the better too, as it provides more meaningful results and meta-analysis may later be applied when data from several comparable studies may be compiled and analysed. Results are only considered to be significant if the likelihood of it occurring by chance is less than 5 per cent. Results are only considered *very* significant if the likelihood of them occurring by chance is less than 1 per cent. It is through trials, more trials and meta-analysis that we have come to the conclusion that HRT is effective for all that it is claimed to be, and that it does exactly what it says it does in its pharmaceutical literature.

So What are the Proven Benefits of HRT?

HRT is currently prescribed because it has been shown repeatedly in clinical trials to alleviate dramatically the uncomfortable symptoms of hot flushes, night sweats and palpitations, because it reverses the changes of vaginal dryness and atrophy, because it helps regulate periods at the time of the menopause, and because it can be useful either on its own or together with other treatments to help urge and stress incontinence. It is currently the gold standard in the prevention of osteoporosis and it has a major role in the prevention of coronary heart disease, especially in women who are at increased risk. But, almost daily, new exciting research is being carried out and published to substantiate the use of HRT in many other clinical settings as well. In themselves these additional benefits may not necessarily mean that it is appropriate for you to begin treatment with HRT. But if other symptoms already exist and you are undecided about the relative pros and cons, knowing about how HRT can affect you in other ways may well persuade you that HRT is or is not for you. Here is a sample of some of the work that has most recently been published.

HRT May Not Increase the Risk of Breast Cancer After All

A large retrospective study from the US Centers for Disease Control and Prevention has failed to find any increase in risk of breast cancer associated with the use of HRT. This flies in the face of earlier research but the study followed nearly 7,000 women for up to 22 years, and its results provide reassurance that any increased relative risk of breast cancer in HRT users must be very small. This is supported by statements made by Professor Michael Baum, a leading breast cancer surgeon in Britain who has criticised the publication of campaign advertisements quoting risks of one in twelve for women dying of breast cancer. He and his colleagues wrote recently in a British medical journal to say that although this figure is technically accurate as a life-time risk, women first have to survive greater threats to their health in order to reach the age of 75 to 80 when the figure applies. 'For most women the lifetime risk of dying of cancer is only one in 26, the other 25 women will die of something else.' The authors of the article went on to say that the association between breast cancer and hormone treatment has been poorly presented. They argued that the risk of dying from breast cancer should be seen in the context of other risks to a woman's life, and pointed out that the risk of dying from heart disease has been seriously under-estimated by women who perceive its threat to be low.

Two further studies, one from Britain and one from Finland, have confirmed common observations that women who develop breast cancer while taking hormone replacement therapy tend to have smaller and less aggressive tumours which are detected earlier and are more easily treated. 'The lower cell proliferation rate and smaller tumour size found in current HRT users suggests a direct inhibitory effect of HRT on the growth of estab-lished breast tumours,' they concluded. The findings did not appear to be related to more frequent mammography screening of such women and the authors of the studies have suggested that further work be done to see whether any direct slowing effect on breast cancer cells occurs as a result of exposure to HRT. One further Swedish study, published in the *British Journal of Cancer* has even suggested that women who were taking HRT before a diagnosis of breast cancer was made may have a prolonged survival rate overall.

HRT Keeps Women Looking Younger

For years devotees of HRT have been saying that they look and feel years younger whilst taking it. Some have even described it as the elixir of eternal youth, and well-known female celebrities have waxed lyrical in a variety of media outlets about the new lease of life HRT has afforded them. Sceptics initially decried such claims and denigrated what they saw as irresponsible commercial salesmanship. Now, however, according to several international studies it looks like HRT really can help to keep women younger looking and shapely. In one study in Germany and another in Santiago in Chile, a panel of men and women were asked to estimate the ages of a hundred white women aged between 35 and 55, from their appearance alone. The estimated ages were then compared with the oestrogen levels as measured in these women's blood tests. Amazingly the results showed that women with a higher oestrogen concentration tended to look younger than their real age, while those with a low oestrogen concentration tended to be rated as older than their real age. The research found that 'the discrepancy between estimated and real age could be as high as eight years in either direction'. How can HRT achieve this? It is probable that HRT increases the amount of collagen (which acts as the scaffolding material holding skin together) within the skin, rendering it thicker, firmer and more elastic. HRT also increases the water content of the skin which, together with increased collagen, reduces the appearance of wrinkles.

HRT Helps Women Retain Their Feminine Shape

It is well known that at the time of the menopause and thereafter many women tend to gain weight as a result of a slower metabolism and a relative deficiency of oestrogen. Italian researchers at the University of Rome compared waist lines and body shape in women who took HRT and those that did not. Both groups of women had similar ages, weights, heights and had given birth to similar numbers of children. Interestingly the waist lines and abdominal fat content of HRT users was found to be significantly smaller than those of women who had never used HRT. So their waist measurements remained smaller and they gained 2.4 times less fat than women who did not take HRT. So much for those common worries that taking HRT makes women gain weight!

HRT Protects Against Alzheimer's Disease

Alzheimer's Disease, a form of dementia, is one of the conditions both men and women worry about as they become older. Research work in the Netherlands has suggested that the risk of Alzheimer's Disease may be reduced by up to 50 per cent in women who use HRT. In particular, the HRT seemed to be especially beneficial when Alzheimer's Disease begins at a comparatively young age, a variant of the condition which has always been thought to be more often genetically rather than environmentally determined.

Other exciting new research is uncovering oestrogen's beneficial effects on brain function. This female hormone not only increases verbal memory throughout the female life span but also appears to protect the brain from the ravages of old age. Oestrogen seems to act as a neural growth factor, influencing the survival, regeneration and ageing of the human brain. This steroidal sex hormone appears to be a powerful antioxidant too, providing brain cells with a chemical shield.

In addition HRT is thought to reduce atherosclerosis, the underlying disorder which leads to hardening of the arteries, thereby increasing blood flow to the brain. Stimulation of message transmission through nerve cell pathways appeared to be enhanced as did the function of chemical transmitters within the brain tissue. HRT also appeared to decrease the deposition of a damaging protein called amyloid when used over a period of time. These studies were given further confirmation from work carried out in Canada on middle-aged women who underwent a surgical menopause. These women found that treatment with oestrogen maintained mental functioning relative to presurgical scores when the ovaries were producing normal amounts of oestrogen, whereas scores of placebo treated women decreased post-operatively. The Canadian researchers concluded that oestrogen specifically improved verbal memory.

Numerous other investigations of women over the age of 65 have consistently shown that those who took oestrogen performed better on neuro-psychological tests of memory compared to age-matched oestrogen non-users. Taken together, these data suggest that hormone replacement therapy may prevent the deterioration in memory that occurs with ageing. Bearing in mind that Alzheimer's Disease alone accounts for up to 60 per cent of cases of dementia, and that memory and concentration problems are commonly reported post-menopausally, these findings are of particular interest. Further well-designed randomised controlled trials will verify whether HRT will be used in the future specifically for the prevention of Alzheimer's Disease.

HRT Might Protect Against Cancer of the Bowel

A report published in the journal *Diseases of the Colon and Rectum* strongly suggested that hormone replacement therapy protected post-menopausal women against colorectal cancer, one of the top three cancer killers overall. The risk of these cancers was lowest among women who were currently taking HRT or who had recently used it, amounting to one third of a reduction compared to the incidence in women who had never used HRT.

HRT Protects Against Heart Disease

Hormone replacement therapy has been shown conclusively to reduce levels of 'bad' cholesterol and to protect against heart disease generally, the single biggest killer of women overall. New work conducted in Holland shows that HRT reduces the levels of a chemical known as homocysteine in the blood, an amino acid linked to the development of cardiovascular disease as well as Alzheimer's Disease. This work noted that the benefits of HRT seemed to be greatest in women with already elevated levels of homocysteine, suggesting that women at greatest risk of developing cardiovascular disease stood to benefit most from taking HRT.

HRT Protects Women Who Smoke from Heart Disease

Researchers in Australia have shown a particular beneficial effect of HRT for post-menopausal women who smoke. As measured by ultrasound tests, smokers who took HRT developed less hardening of their artery walls, their arteries remained more elastic and, in addition, their 'bad' cholesterol levels were lowered. It appears that women who smoke therefore derive particular benefit from HRT.

HRT Does Not Just Benefit Women Who are Already Healthy

It was once thought that HRT's benefits have been overstated because women who take it are thought to be highly motivated, well educated and enjoy healthy lifestyles anyway. New work carried out on HRT users measured and compared the effect of medium and low doses of HRT on the incidence of hip fractures and heart attacks. Researchers found that there was better protection against the fractures and the heart disease in women who used a medium rather than just a low dose of HRT. Since this effectively circumnavigates the problem of the 'healthy user effect' it highlights very nicely the relative benefits.

HRT Preserves Muscle Strength

A relatively common symptom of the menopause is weakness and fatigue. The ability to move the thumb across the front of the palm and bring it into contact with the fingers is an essential evolutionary adaptation of the human hand, and British researchers measured muscle strength in the muscle largely responsible for such movements, the adductor pollicis muscle. This muscle is essential for many everyday tasks from the relatively gross movements required to grip doorknobs and open screw top jars and bottles, to finer two-handed actions such as dealing with small buttons and tying shoelaces. The study showed that HRT was capable of increasing isometric muscle strength in post-menopausal women by as much as 15 per cent, a result corroborated by other similar studies carried out since.

HRT Improves Sex Life After the Menopause

According to a recent US survey, taking HRT is likely to increase satisfaction with your sex life. The survey conducted by Yankelovich Partners Inc. found that 82 per cent of HRT users said their sex lives were as good as or better than before the menopause, compared with 69 per cent of women not using HRT. More than half the women reported thinking more about sex than ten years previously, and 43 per cent felt their sexual desires had not diminished since their thirties. This greater enjoyment of sex in middle age was attributed to having less responsibility to rear children, a reduced fear of unwanted pregnancy, being happy at work and having financial security. Interestingly, 80 per cent of women surveyed said they felt more independent and in control of their lives since their menopause, and more than 87 per cent reported feeling a positive attitude towards it.

HRT May Help Prevent Parkinson's Disease

A small but significant study carried out at the Mayo clinic in the US suggested a link between oestrogen deficiency and Parkinson's Disease. It had previously been noticed that women who had had a hysterectomy had a three-fold risk of Parkinson's Disease compared to women who had not. The researchers then compared women in Olmstead County who developed Parkinson's Disease over a 15-year period with women of the same age group who did not. Those who developed Parkinson's tended not to have used HRT.

HRT Can Prevent Periodontal Disease

Loss of bone mineral density, which occurs in osteoporosis, may contribute quite significantly towards tooth loss and periodontal disease. As HRT remains the best treatment for the prevention of such processes it clearly has a benefit in dentistry.

HRT Remains the Number One Choice for the Prevention of Osteoporosis

According to new evidence-based guidelines produced by the Royal College of Physicians, HRT remains the preferred therapy for the prevention and treatment of osteoporosis. Other strategies for decreasing fracture risk for post-menopausal women, such as increasing the level of physical activity, reducing smoking and increasing dietary calcium intake, cannot be nearly as effective because there is no actual evidence the strategy would have any impact and is therefore not considered reliable enough by the Royal College of Physicians. Instead they say, 'HRT prevents bone loss and decreases the risk of fragility fractures. Giving HRT for periods of up to ten years would yield significant benefit with minimised risk.'

HRT Can Benefit Ethnic Minority Groups if Only the Message can be Conveyed

The results of a south London survey conducted by Dr Tess Harris and colleagues at St George's Hospital, London, and published in the *British Medical Journal* reveal that women from the Caribbean, West Africa and the Indian sub-continent were much less likely than white women to use HRT and were therefore missing opportunities for health screening and health promotion. Better education and targeting of such populations will obviously help.

HRT Will Benefit More Women When it is Better Understood

In the United States, less than a third of post-menopausal women currently receive HRT and the proportion is probably very similar in Britain. Even in those that do take HRT some 20–30 per cent never get as far as taking their prescription to the chemist, and a similar proportion discontinue their HRT within six to eight months. This is a shame because it is ignorance and confusion about how HRT works and how any short-term side effects may be overcome that accounts for many of these difficulties. Better motivation amongst health care professionals, and better understanding and knowledge within the community mean that many thousands more women could take advantage of the many benefits discussed above.

Summing Up the Benefits

Women who are at high risk of heart disease, strokes, osteoporosis and possibly Alzheimer's Disease will gain the most benefit from the long-term protection against these conditions that HRT provides. Also, those women whose periods cease earlier than the average because of an early natural menopause or because of hysterectomy or illness are particularly advised to take HRT. Hormone replacement therapy can start at any time after menopausal symptoms begin and even many years after the menopause. To achieve maximum benefit HRT should begin as close to the menopause as possible, however. It should be taken for two to three years for symptomatic relief, since we know that in most cases hot flushes will not return after such a duration provided the dose of HRT is tailed off gradually. HRT should continue for at least five to ten years, however, to provide protection against fractures, heart disease and strokes. Remember that HRT is not a contraceptive so women beginning treatment before the menopause should continue using effective contraception (see page 125). Overall the most common form of HRT is to combine continuous oestrogens with a monthly course of progestogens, although women who have had a hysterectomy and who do not need to protect the lining of their womb with progestogen can take oestrogen therapy alone.

CHAPTER 14

HORMONE REPLACEMENT THERAPY – THE SIDE EFFECTS AND RISKS

The benefits of any treatment must always be weighed against its risks. We have seen in previous chapters that the potential benefits of HRT are considerable and numerous and women now have at their disposal over 50 different types of HRT enabling them to tailor therapy to their individual and specific needs. However, it is also vital, as it is throughout the entire field of medicine, that treatments are looked at from the point of view of the potential risk as well as the potential benefit. In recent years carefully designed scientific research, incorporating very large numbers of women, have provided us with information about the pros and cons of HRT, and careful reporting of any adverse events has allowed us to detect any side effects, even very rare ones such as those which occur in one in every 10,000 or more patients. In other words, modern medicine has given us sophisticated and reliable methods of assessing the balance of benefit against risk for HRT. A full list of the side effects of oestrogens, progestogens and testosterone HRT is given below, and amongst them can be found the commonest problems, which regrettably influence a relatively high proportion of women into discontinuing their HRT within the first few months of treatment. In addition, the main serious concerns of women who are offered HRT include the risk of breast cancer or blood clots as a result of taking it. Hopefully the following pages will put these side effects and risks into a proper perspective.

SIDE EFFECTS OF OESTROGENS, PROGESTOGENS AND METHYLTESTOSTERONE

	Oestrogens	Progestogens	Androgens (Methyltestosterone)
Thromboembolic phenomena (blood clots)	Thrombophlebitis pulmonary embolism	Thrombophlebitis pulmonary embolism	
Genito-urinary	Breakthrough bleeding, spotting, increased uterine fibroid size, cervical secretion change, lighter or absent periods, endometrial and ovarian cancer	Breakthrough bleeding, spotting, cervical secretion change, lighter or absent periods	Cessation of periods, menstrual irregularities clitoral enlargement
Breast	Tenderness, enlargement, breast cancer	Tenderness, nipple discharge	
Gastro-intestinal	Nausea, abdominal cramps, bloating, jaundice, gallbladder disease	Nausea, jaundice, bloating	Nausea, jaundice and hepatitis, alterations in liver function tests, liver cancer
Skin	Patchy skin pigmentation, skin rashes, loss of scalp hair	Urticaria, acne, hair loss, unwanted hair	Unwanted hair, male pattern of baldness, acne
Eyes	Steepening of corneal curvature, intolerance of contact lenses, retinal vascular lesions	Retinal thrombosis, visual disturbance (optic neuritis)	
Nervous system	Headache, migraine, dizziness mental depression	Insomnia, headache, mood swings, depression, PMS	Headache, anxiety, depression
Miscellaneous	Weight change, reduced carbohydrate tolerance, oedema, libido changes	Weight change, oedema	Hypercalcemia, oedema

COMMON TRANSIENT PROBLEMS CAUSED BY HRT

Irregular Bleeding with HRT

One of the main reasons why 20–30 per cent of women discontinue their HRT in the first few months of treatment, despite obtaining certain benefits, is because of irregular bleeding. The majority feel that they had been looking forward to having no periods after the menopause and regard the withdrawal bleeds which they experience on HRT as either unnatural or simply inconvenient. Those who are offered bleed-free forms of HRT may find themselves entirely satisfied with this alternative, although breakthrough bleeding can still remain a problem, particularly in younger women or in women who are not 12 months beyond the menopause. Women who take cyclical preparations should expect to experience bleeding at a regular time every month with the vast majority, say 90 per cent of women, falling into this category. Remember, however, that the occurrence of bleeding may vary between preparations. Total absence of bleeding will occur in a small proportion of women, up to 10 per cent, and requires no further investigations providing menopausal symptoms are under control. Irregular bleeding, however, should be investigated and referral considered if no cause can be found, such as failure to take the HRT at the right times. Women on long cycle HRT (see page 281) will expect four bleeds a year, but these preparations may cause initial irregular bleeding in a few women within the first two cycles, although this tends to settle. Investigation is generally advised if this irregular bleeding persists for more than the first six months (two quarterly cycles). In continuous combined HRT preparations (see page 283), light bleeding and/or spotting is common in the first three to six months of treatment, but if pelvic discomfort or heavy bleeding occurs during this time further investigation is required. Similarly, if bleeding persists or starts after these initial six months, again investigation and referral is recommended.

To summarise, any woman presenting with irregular bleeding

should be asked about whether she is taking her HRT in the right way. If she has had any vomiting or severe diarrhoea recently this could be affecting her absorption of HRT through her digestive system. She should be asked if she is taking any other medication which might be altering the metabolism of her HRT within her liver. Women should be referred for further tests if vaginal bleeding is excessive or particularly uncomfortable, if it occurs after six months of continuous combined HRT, if it occurs after a prolonged initial duration of no periods in women taking continuous combined HRT, or if the bleeding becomes much heavier when initially it was very light and perfectly acceptable.

Weight Gain

Fear of putting on weight is one of the commonest reasons women cite for refusing the offer of HRT. It is also a common reason why some women choose to discontinue their HRT within the first few months. However, there is growing evidence to suggest that these women should be strongly reassured that, if anything, their HRT is likely to help them to prevent further weight gain. Several scientific studies have shown that women gain weight after the menopause because of relative oestrogen deficiency and because of an increased influence of testosterone secreted by their ovaries at this time of their life. In addition, any weight they put on tends to be distributed in the male pattern, that is, around the waist and abdomen and away from the hips and thighs, which is the traditional area for weight gain in premenopausal women. Recent studies carried out in Italy showed very clearly that weight gain was 2.4 times less in women taking HRT than in women who did not take HRT, and that any weight gain reported tended to be distributed in the female distribution around the hips and thighs. It should also be remembered that much of the weight gain which occurs after the menopause is age-related. The metabolism of the body slows with increasing years and exercise levels tend to diminish, so that women eating the same diet that they have always enjoyed will burn up less of these calories despite leading similar lifestyles. Some doctors have attempted to help women on HRT who are worried about weight gain by changing the type of preparation they are using, or by prescribing diuretics (water tablets) in addition. Whilst trying a different formulation of HRT to overcome problems is reasonable, extra prescriptions for more medication are not generally recommended.

Nausea

The oestrogen component of HRT may certainly cause some nausea initially. The effect tends to wear off but for a small proportion of women it can be a persistent and inconvenient problem. Sometimes simply taking HRT tablets with meals or last thing at night is all that is required. Starting on a lower dose and then increasing this later is another useful trick. If nausea persists, however, for more than two to three cycles, it may be better to abandon the synthetic oestrogens used in tablets and revert to skin patches which supply a lower overall dose.

Breast Tenderness

Some women notice some breast tenderness when they initially take HRT and understandably worry that this may have some sinister cause. They have heard alarmist stories about the risk of breast cancer and they may regard any discomfort as an abnormal sign. In fact breast tenderness in itself is rarely associated with breast cancer. Furthermore, this side effect, like that of nausea, usually disappears spontaneously within the first few weeks of treatment. When it is uncomfortable, however, reducing salt intake and cutting out tea and coffee may help, as will the use of a supportive bra such as a sports bra. Vitamin B6 and evening primrose oil supplements are well worth a try too.

Side Effects Due to Particular Formulations of HRT

Some side effects are experienced with certain preparations of HRT but not others. For example, nausea is more common with

HRT in tablet form. Irregular bleeding in women taking continuous combined HRT is more commonly seen in younger women and those not far enough beyond the menopause. Skin patches, on the other hand, are capable of causing local skin irritation and implants may leave tiny scars or even become infected around the wound. This is most likely to occur after testosterone implants but any implant can push towards the surface and sometimes even be expelled spontaneously. Even vaginal HRT is capable of stimulating the lining of the womb, leading to endometrial hyperplasia when it is used for some time in high dose and when it has not been opposed by using a progestogen. Sexual partners might also notice side-effects if such vaginal HRT has been used as a sexual lubricant.

Common Transient Side Effects of Progestogens

Side effects often attributed to the progestogens include premenstrual syndrome, breast tenderness, mood swings, depression, weight gain, bloating, headaches and acne. Combined HRT makes use of two main forms of progestogens, mainly the C19 family which is more closely related to testosterone, and the newer C21 group of progestogens. It is the C19 forms, namely norethisterone, norgestrel and levo-norgestrel, which have the reputation for causing most side effects, whereas the C21 group, namely medroxy progesterone acetate or dydrogesterone are said to be better tolerated. Sometimes women with progestogen-like side effects will be changed from a preparation containing a C19 progestogen to one containing a C21 progestogen, although another option is to use a combined HRT patch which employs a smaller dose of hormone overall. Recently there have been additional choices made available, one of which includes an inter-uterine device which releases small amounts of progestogen over a long period of time. If this is being used for contraception anyway the use of continuous oestrogens simultaneously provides an effective regime for HRT with minimal side effects. A vaginal gel containing natural progesterone (Crinone) may also be considered as part of HRT.

MORE SERIOUS CONCERNS

Cancer of the Breast

Many women have been hugely influenced by adverse publicity in the media linking HRT to the development of breast cancer. Whilst thousands of column inches have been devoted to high-lighting this perceived risk, the benefits of HRT in protecting against heart disease and osteoporosis, from which many more women will ultimately die, has been understated. How can we keep the truth about breast cancer and HRT in perspective? In June 1997 a leading cancer specialist, Professor Michael Baum, was reported as saying, 'It is possible to have too much cancer awareness' (see page 157.)

HRT is considered by many who have benefited from it, and by experts who have studied its authentic development since the 1920s, to be the most important preventative medicine in the twentieth century. Perhaps one of the reasons why only about 15 per cent of eligible women in Britain use it properly is because they have been so scared by alarmist reporting. Again, Professor Michael Baum and colleagues John Bunker and Joan Houghton have attempted to put this risk of breast cancer in perspective in an article published in the *British Medical Journal* in 1998. Again, they refer to the risk of one in 12 women dying from breast cancer by saying that women first have to survive greater threats to their health in order to reach the age of 75 to 80 when the figure applies. 'For most women the lifetime risk of dying of breast cancer is only one in 26, the other 25 women will die of some-thing else.' Younger women in fact face a much smaller risk of breast cancer with only one in 625 women under the age of 35 in England and Wales developing it and only one in 56 by the age of 50. Even then the risk depends on other factors such as obesity, alcohol consumption and family history of the disease. The authors argued that the risk of dying from breast cancer should be seen in the context of other risks to a woman's life: 'The risk of dying from heart disease has been under-estimated by women and its threat perceived to be low.'

Attempts have, of course, been made to quantify the risk of women who take HRT developing breast cancer. The biggest ever scientific review, which looked at all available evidence on the subject, suggested a very slight increase in the number of breast cancers diagnosed in women who use HRT than in those who did not. This meta-analysis of several large studies collated from all around the world by independent experts has been widely accepted and endorsed. It showed that using HRT for a short time-span around the menopause hardly affects a woman's risk of breast cancer at all. For women aged 50 not using HRT there would in any case be about 45 in every 1,000 who will have breast cancer diagnosed before they reach the age of 70. The study showed that the extra number of breast cancer cases found in women who do use HRT, over and above the 45 occurring in women in this age group anyway, has been estimated by researchers as follows:

Length of time on HRT	Extra breast cancers over 20 years
5 years' use	2 per 1,000 women
10 years' use	6 per 1,000 women
15 years' use	12 per 1,000 women

These statistics show that there are clearly quantifiable, albeit small, risks in taking HRT since it slightly increases the risk of breast cancer. The extra chance of developing breast cancer beyond your age group disappears about two years after stopping HRT in any event. Women must weigh up the risks against the benefits. Bearing in mind Professor Baum's remarks about the lifetime risk of breast cancer, remember that all women face a one in four risk of having a heart attack, and a one in three risk of having a fracture linked to thinning bones. For the majority of women, therefore, the benefits of taking HRT greatly outweigh the risks. Of course much will depend upon a woman's own personal circumstances, because if she has a strong family history of breast cancer and has other risk factors this needs to be borne in mind. On the other hand, if she has a strong family history of heart disease or many risk factors for osteoporosis, against which HRT is highly protective, this too should sway her decision. (See the risk factor chart on page 306.) As with other aspects of HRT, the pros and cons should be discussed with the health care professionals involved.

Interestingly, the very latest research emanating from the United States Centers for Disease Control and Prevention, conducted on nearly 7,000 women over a period of 22 years suggested that there is *no* increase in breast cancer risk with HRT, a study which provides ample reassurance that any increased relative risk of breast cancer in HRT users suggested by other studies must be very small. Furthermore, a Swedish study published in the *British Journal of Cancer* in 1999 even suggested that HRT used by women before their diagnosis of breast cancer was made may actually prolong survival. Such women had a significantly better outlook than women who didn't take HRT and this is thought to be because the tumours which did arise were smaller, less aggressive in their behaviour, less likely to spread to other parts of the body, were detected earlier and more easily and responded better to treatment. The researchers were of the opinion that HRT appeared to slow down tumour growth. The question was raised of whether more frequent mammography in the HRT users could have accounted for these findings, but although mammography screening was also associated with longer survival, there was no evidence that HRT users were in fact screened any more frequently than the women who never used HRT.

Clearly these more recent findings are extremely encouraging and there is obviously a need to remain cautious about statistics relating to survival from breast cancer when they are used within the popular media. When a television programme or magazine article states that 'a woman's risk increases by 2 per cent for every year of using HRT' this does not mean that women on HRT have two times the risk, that is, double the risk of developing a problem. Yet many members of the public take it to mean this. There is a vast difference between 2 per cent and a doubling. Similarly a newspaper headline which states that 'women run a 30 per cent increase in risk' does not mean that 30 per cent of women who use HRT will develop a problem. The words 'increase in risk' must be carefully interpreted in view of what the original risk was in the first place. In much the same way, if an NHS nurse is informed by the Government that she or he can be thrilled to expect a 10 per cent increase in salary, whilst it may initially sound marvellous, a statistician can soon bring her or him down to earth again by pointing out that 10 per cent of a tiny salary in the first place is not very much!

Deep Vein Thrombosis (DVT)

Blood clots which form in the deep veins of the lower legs generally pose a small risk to women whether or not they take HRT. In a group of 10,000 women not taking HRT only one would be expected to develop a DVT in the future. If 10,000 similar women all took HRT, statistics show that three would be likely to develop a DVT in the future. To put matters in perspective, however, in normal pregnancy the risk increases to six out of 10,000 women. Also, any additional risk is only present during the first year of taking the HRT and not thereafter.

The clinical significance of a deep vein thrombosis is that the blood clot which forms in the leg veins can become dislodged, travelling upwards in the venous circulation towards the heart and lungs. A pulmonary embolus occurs when a blood clot ends up blocking the major arteries to the lungs, whereas if a blood clot ends up blocking the arterial supply to the brain, a stroke may result. Very occasionally these events prove fatal and therefore the very slightly increased risk of a deep vein thrombosis in the first year of using HRT should be considered. This is especially true of women who have a past personal history of venous thrombosis or a strong family history, and those women who are overweight, immobilised or who have severe varicose veins in which the blood flow is relatively stagnant and much more likely to clot anyway. Modern diagnostic techniques have shown that these women, as well as women who smoke cigarettes, are overall running a higher risk of experiencing blood clotting problems.

Cancer of the Womb (Endometrial Cancer)

In the earliest pioneering days of HRT treatment oestrogen was used on its own, which led to the proliferation of endometrial cells. Since the influence of progesterone was absent in these post-menopausal women it led to overstimulation of the endometrium and an increased risk of development of cancerous changes. It was soon discovered that up to a four-fold increase in the risk of endometrial cancer was the result. As it happened, the survival rate of this type of malignancy was very high, being 99 per cent at five years, but the risk of developing the cancer increased with every year that the oestrogen was used. Thankfully, doctors found that by using progestogen in addition to the oestrogen, to create a 'period' at the end of each treatment cycle, this problem could be avoided. It is now known that an adequate dose and duration of treatment with a progestogen can reduce the risks of endometrial cancer to the same of that of women who do not use HRT, and even possibly lower than that.

Cancer of the Ovary and Cervix

Although these cancers are more common overall than endometrial cancer, there is no evidence that HRT alters the risk of these cancers developing. There is therefore no reason not to take HRT if a woman is worried about these cancers developing, nor in fact does HRT necessarily need to be withheld even if these cancers are already present.

Which Women Should Not Take HRT?

There is a small proportion of women who should specifically not take HRT, because in their individual situation it would pose a greater risk to their health than if they did not take it. There is also a small proportion of women who are eligible for treatment but in whom it should be used with considerable caution. Finally, there are a number of women who have pre-existing medical conditions who have been led to believe that they are not suitable for HRT, whereas in actual fact they would be perfectly safe taking it. See box.

CONTRA-INDICATIONS (conditions in which HRT should NOT be used)	**CAUTION** (conditions in which HRT should be used with considerable caution)
Breast cancer	Gallstones
Endometrial cancer	Fibroids
Acute liver disease	Endometriosis
Undiagnosed vaginal bleeding	Benign breast lumps
	Strong family history of breast cancer
Active thrombosis	Strong family history of thrombosis
Pregnancy	Migraine headaches
	Epilepsy
	Obesity with a BMI more than 30kg per sq m
	Multiple sclerosis
	Otosclerosis

Each of these conditions and the interaction with HRT warrants further explanation.

Breast Cancer

Because breast cancer may in some cases be influenced by the oestrogen contained within HRT it cannot be recommended as a treatment in this condition. This is still the most cautious approach at present, although with new research coming through (see page 248) it looks as if the possible association between HRT and breast cancer may appear to have been over-emphasised. Some specialist gynaecologists have in fact prescribed HRT for women who have already had breast cancer treatment in the past, where their severe menopausal symptoms and their increased risks of heart disease and osteoporosis make the overall benefit of taking the HRT outweigh the risk.

Endometrial Cancer

The effect of unopposed oestrogen on endometrial cells is well documented. Combined HRT, where oestrogen is opposed by progestogen, eradicates the risk of endometrial cancer but whilst there is little strong evidence to suggest that women who have already been successfully treated for cancer of the womb should not take HRT, there remains a theoretical risk that any remaining cancer cells could flare up again.

Acute Liver Disease

If liver disease is only mild and blood tests reveal that liver function is normal, HRT may still be taken. But in more severe cases, where liver function is abnormal, HRT is contra-indicated. This is because HRT in tablet form is absorbed straight through the intestine to the liver before it reaches the bloodstream. If the liver were already diseased this would create problems for an already overloaded liver. In cases of mild liver disease where HRT is recommended, a non-oral form of HRT, such as patch therapy, would be more appropriate as the hormone finds its way directly into the bloodstream without first having to negotiate the liver.

Undiagnosed Vaginal Bleeding

Whenever unusual vaginal bleeding is reported HRT should be held back until the cause has been identified. Usually there is a straightforward explanation but it would be wrong to prescribe HRT where possible endometrial cancer exists.

Active Thrombosis

If a woman is suffering from a proven venous thrombosis clearly HRT should not be prescribed as it might exacerbate the condition.

Pregnancy

Nobody would prescribe HRT in pregnancy, but since this is the most common reason for a woman's periods to stop, and since pregnancy sometimes occurs even in the late forties, that small chance should always be excluded before HRT is commenced.

Gallstones

The oestrogens in HRT are broken down by the liver and then excreted in the urine. Parts of these steroid molecules find their way to the gallbladder where they can increase the likelihood of gallstones, leading to abdominal pain and jaundice. HRT should therefore be used carefully by any women who have had gallstones in the past unless, of course, they have had their gallbladder removed (cholecystectomy).

Fibroids

These benign growths in the muscular wall of the uterus are sensitive to oestrogen. Many women approaching their menopause can look forward to their symptoms spontaneously improving as their fibroids become smaller as their oestrogen levels fall. If HRT is started these fibroids can enlarge again, causing heavy or irregular bleeding or a feeling of abdominal swelling. Sometimes when a woman is examined internally before commencing HRT, fibroids may be discovered by the examining doctor. If this is the case and the fibroids are small HRT may be started, although a repeat check should be made within a few months to assess any change in the size of the fibroids. These days regular ultrasound scanning is a preferable and accurate alternative. Any woman who has had a hysterectomy because of fibroids can certainly take HRT, and because she no longer has a womb she can take oestrogen-only HRT without the need for a progestogen.

Endometriosis

Since endometrial tissue is stimulated by oestrogen, there is always the small possibility that endometriosis can start up again and cause symptoms after the menopause when HRT is prescribed. This happens only in about 5 per cent of cases so a decision as to whether to prescribe HRT or not must be based on the benefit against risk ratio. There are, of course, alternatives to standard HRT, such as tibolone, which would overcome this problem and help menopausal symptoms at the same time.

Benign Breast Lumps

If benign breast disease is diagnosed before HRT is started, there is a very slightly increased risk of breast cancer developing if the HRT is continued for more than ten years. However, if the benign breast disease develops after starting HRT there appears to be no such increased risk.

Strong Family History of Breast Cancer

If one or more first degree relatives have a history of breast cancer this will statistically increase the chance of a woman developing breast cancer herself, in which case HRT should be used with caution.

Strong Family History of Thrombo Embolism

If other close relatives have had a strong history of blood clots or the consequences of blood clots, such as pulmonary embolism or strokes, there will be a statistically higher chance of a woman developing them herself and she should only use HRT with caution.

Migraine Headaches

Migraine headaches can be made more serious or more frequent as a result of taking HRT. If this proves to be the case after a reasonable trial period, withdrawal of hormone replacement therapy becomes appropriate. An alternative is to consider taking other preventative treatments for migraine, in addition to HRT, although a full discussion with your doctor would be required.

Epilepsy

Since it is known that epileptic seizures may be triggered by ovulation and by menstruation, there is a clear link between higher levels of oestrogen and convulsions. On the other hand, progesterone appears to reduce the frequency of seizures by up to 50 per cent. More work needs to be carried out to assess the importance of HRT in this condition, but for the time being HRT should be used very carefully in the presence of epilepsy.

Obesity With a Body Mass Index More Than 30kg per sq m (see page 69)

Being overweight is associated with a number of different factors which may impinge on the safety of HRT. It should therefore be used with caution if obesity is present.

Multiple Sclerosis

The response of women with multiple sclerosis to a prescription for HRT is unpredictable. Some women appear to notice an improvement in their symptoms whereas others may notice deterioration. Again, this is a situation where the benefits must be weighed against the possible risks.

Otosclerosis

This inherited disorder impairs hearing due to hardening of the tiny bones within the middle ear cavity. In some women HRT leads to a permanent deterioration in the condition.

Drug Interactions

Occasionally HRT may interfere with other medication used in a variety of medical conditions. Therefore women being treated for an overactive thyroid gland, for asthma, or for epilepsy should check with their doctor before considering this therapy.

Miscellaneous

Some women may be affected by a number of rarer conditions including porphyria, kidney conditions, heart disorders and Roter Syndrome and they should check with their doctors to assess their suitability for HRT.

When Should HRT be Stopped Immediately?

Occasionally a woman taking HRT is unable to contact her doctor or practice nurse urgently when she has pressing questions about whether or not she should continue with her treatment. The *Monthly Index of Medical Specialities* lists the following reasons for immediate discontinuation of treatment.

- If any migraine-type headaches begin for the first time.
- If frequent severe headaches or acute visual disturbances are noticed.
- If there are any signs of blood clotting, including breathlessness or coughing blood, or any jaundice.
- If there is any chance that pregnancy has occurred in a woman taking HRT.

MOST WOMEN CAN BENEFIT FROM HRT

Although the above list seems lengthy there are in fact few women overall who are unable to take HRT on medical grounds. Generally speaking, when HRT is prescribed appropriately there are few risks linked with it. What is more, many women who are in fact eligible to take HRT have been unfortunately steered away from it or made very anxious about taking it because of conditions which were once thought to put them at increased risk, but now are not. Diabetics, for example, can take HRT provided their blood glucose control is fairly stable, and there are positive reasons why women with raised blood pressure and women who smoke *should* take HRT.

There are good reasons now why women who are already on HRT but who have had a heart attack should continue to take their HRT, as it offers them protection against another heart attack; even women who have had a previous deep vein thrombosis may be prescribed HRT, provided they have no blood disorder putting them at permanent increased risk of a thrombosis. They would, however, be advised to take their HRT in non-oral forms.

Lastly, unlike the oral contraceptive pill which should be strictly discontinued four to six weeks before any surgical operation is carried out, it is less important that HRT is stopped as it has far less of a potential to cause thrombosis. However, in the *Monthly Index of Medical Specialities*, the doctors' standard guide to commonly prescribed drugs in the UK, women on HRT are still advised to discontinue HRT for any future planned (elective) surgery.

Minimising Risks

Most women who take HRT understand the concept of benefit and risk. Armed with the correct information they can sensibly make their own decision about whether to take HRT and what is the best formulation for them. There is much that can be done to minimise any possible side effects. The dose of hormone may be kept to a minimum and provided the menopausal symptoms, for which the HRT was prescribed in the first place, are controlled the lower the dose the better. However, there would be a minimum necessary dose of progestogen required to oppose the oestrogen and protect the lining of the womb from being overstimulated and leading to endometrial hyperplasia or cancer. Furthermore, if side effects are experienced, a different type of delivery may provide just as much relief from symptoms but without side effects. Patches may well fulfil this goal when used instead of tablets. It is also worth considering changing the type of progestogen used in any type of HRT. Some of the newer C21 type of progestogens, for example, are associated with many fewer side effects than the C19 group of progestogens. Remember, too, that in the vast majority of cases any minor side effects experienced tend to settle completely within three to four months of being on HRT. This is because it takes a little while for your body to readjust to the hormone changes again, just as it did during the natural menopause. So try not to be one of the 20–30 per cent of women who discontinue their HRT within the first few months because of initial problems. There is generally always one type of formulation which will suit every single woman and, with a little help from your doctor or your specialist, you should be able to find the one which broadly satisfies all your requirements without causing problems. Do be realistic, however: there is no such thing as the elixir of eternal youth, and no medication is entirely free of side effects, especially if it was never used appropriately in the first place.

Check-Ups

There is much debate about how women taking HRT should be monitored by their doctors. Women, of course, can be taking their HRT for lots of different reasons. Some will be perfectly healthy women who are only taking HRT to prevent symptoms like hot flushes and night sweats. Others will have important risk factors for osteoporosis or heart disease and they will be seeing their GP for these problems anyway. Another group of women will be seeing their gynaecologist, endocrinologist or other specialists as part of their hospital follow-up for conditions such as hysterectomy or hormonal problems. Specialist menopause clinics, however, are regrettably few and far between and remain unavailable to the majority of women in Britain.

The current recommended approach is a 'shared care' one as proposed by the Royal College of Obstetricians and Gynaecologists, the Royal College of General Practitioners and the National Osteoporosis Society. This calls for the regular monitoring of women who have had an early hysterectomy and need long-term treatment with HRT. For other women on HRT, however, probably the best policy is simply to find a family doctor who has a special interest in HRT. This is important because there have been many advances and refinements in HRT over recent years and, with the best will in the world, busy GPs with so much to try to keep abreast of find it difficult to keep bang up to date with the latest therapeutic advances.

Overall it is good practice to check a woman's personal medical history and family history, particularly focusing on areas which may contra-indicate the use of HRT or require further investigation. Family doctors should provide lifestyle guidance along with balanced counselling to supplement advice provided with patient information leaflets. A woman's blood pressure and weight should be taken as a base line before she commences on HRT, and all doctors should advise about breast awareness and check on a woman's entry into the National Breast Screening Programme. Sometimes it will be appropriate to examine a woman's breasts and a cervical smear should be taken at the times dictated by the cervical screening programme, and at other times too if appropriate. Occasionally a pelvic examination will be carried out if any symptoms are present.

Initially a three-month supply of HRT should be issued and it would be a wonderful ideal if the recipient could be given a contact telephone number, either to the doctor or to his or her practice nurse, in case any problems arose within that time. Unfortunately this rarely happens in practice. Thereafter a check-up three months later to discuss any side effects, to assess the bleeding pattern established with the HRT, and to talk about how easy or difficult it is for the patient to take the HRT correctly, is extremely helpful. Following that an appointment after six months and then every year, when this process is repeated, represents sound medical practice.

CHAPTER 15

DIFFERENT TYPES OF HRT

Listening to people talking about HRT you might easily get the impression that there is only one type. You are either taking it or you are not. It will either suit you or it will not. It will give you side effects or it will not. But there are a large number of different types of HRT now available and many options from which to choose. You may have your own preferences if, for example, you are keener on a natural hormone rather than a synthetic one. You will find that you are more likely to notice side effects on one preparation rather than another. Some of you will not respond very quickly to HRT tablets because for various reasons you do not absorb the hormones very readily by that route, whereas you can obtain considerable relief from your menopausal symptoms by taking HRT in another form, such as a skin patch.

The response to HRT is a very individual thing and that is why each of you must be treated as an individual by your doctor so that your unique needs and wishes are satisfied. Unfortunately, because there is still far too little knowledge about the different types of hormones used and formulations in which they are packaged, a relatively high percentage (up to 30 per cent) of women initially treated with HRT discontinue their treatment within the first six months. This is a great shame as there are considerable benefits to be had, not just in the short term but for many years to come in terms of prevention against osteoporosis and heart disease, for example. That is why understanding about all the different types of HRT and how it should be taken is so important.

Do You Still Have a Womb?

In the early days of hormone replacement therapy oestrogen alone was used and was given for three out of every four weeks, a withdrawal bleed occurring in the last few days. However, over the course of time it became apparent that stimulation of the lining of the womb (the endometrium) led in some women to cellular changes which increased the risk of the development of endometrial cancer. This type of oestrogen-only hormone therapy was proved to double any existing risk. For this reason, only women who have had a hysterectomy (and therefore no longer have an endometrium) should now use oestrogen-only HRT, and all other women whose wombs remain intact should use oestrogen combined with a progestogen which effectively balances out the proliferative effects of the oestrogen on the endometrial cells. This 'combined' HRT protects against the development of any increased risk of endometrial cancer and it is also a more logical approach as there is a relative deficiency of progesterone after the menopause as well as a deficiency of oestrogen anyway.

Different Oestrogens

As we saw in Chapter 13, the oestrogens used in HRT are either natural in that they are very similar in structure and effects to the oestrogens produced by your body, or synthetic in that they also produce similar effects to natural oestrogens but have a significantly different structure. The natural varieties include oestradiol, oestrone, oestriol, equilin and 17 alpha-dihydroequilin. The synthetic forms include ethinyloestradiol, dienoestrol and mestranol. On the whole the natural oestrogens are recommended for HRT as they tend to have fewer side effects. The synthetic oestrogens, being more potent, are generally used more often for contraception because they are powerful enough to prevent ovulation. All oestrogens may be available as tablets, patches, implants or gels for absorption into the whole of the body, or as vaginal creams, pessaries, tablets or rings for use in the vagina only.

Different Progestogens

Since progesterone, the naturally produced female sex hormone, is so easily broken down in tablet form, it would have to be given either in impractical repeated dosages throughout the day or in suppository form, either of which is unacceptable to the majority of women. Instead, synthetic types of progesterone, where the chemical structure has been subtly altered, are used as these *are* effective as tablets or as skin patches. These synthetic forms of progesterone are known as progestogens. Figure 22 summarises the different forms of oestrogen and progestogen preparations.

Figure 22

Forms of oestrogen and progestogen preparations

Oestrogen	Progestogen
Tablets – oral	Tablets – oral
Patch	Combined with oestrogen in patches
Implant	
Gel	
Cream	
Pessary	
Vaginal ring	

Tablets

Usually HRT is prescribed in tablet form. If you have had a hysterectomy you only require oestrogen treatment since you do not need the effect of progestogen to protect the lining of the womb against endometrial cancer. Your oestrogen tablets should be taken on a daily basis without a break and roughly at the same time each day. There are many different commercial brands of these tablets available on prescription, containing different forms of oestrogen. Some contain a fixed dose in each tablet, whereas others are designed to mirror the menstrual cycle

284 *A Change for the Better*

more closely by adjusting the dose in the tablets in each 28-day course. See Figure 23.

Figure 23

Oestrogen-only HRT Tablets

Brand	Oestrogen	Dose
Climaval	Oestradiol Valerate	1mg (grey-blue) 2mg (blue)
Elleste Solo	Oestradiol	1mg (white) 2mg (orange)
Harmogen	Oestrone	0.93mg (peach)
Harmonin	Oestriol/Oestradiol/ Oestrone	0.27mg/0.6mg/ 1.4mg (pink)
Ovestin	Oestriol	1mg (white)
Premarin	Conjugated oestrogens	0.625mg (maroon) 1.25mg (yellow) 2.5mg (purple)
Progynova	Oestradiol	1mg (beige) 2mg (blue)
Zumenon	Oestradiol	1mg (white) 2mg (orange)

The majority of women have not had a hysterectomy as they approach their menopause and when they are prescribed HRT, along with their continuous oestrogen, they will need to take a course of progestogen tablets every month for about 10 to 14 days. To make complying with the prescription easier, calendar packs combine the progestogen tablets with the oestrogen tablets. This is known as 'sequential combined HRT'. Occasionally, you may want to make your own choices about which oestrogen you want to take and there may be no ready calendar pack which suits you. Equally, specialist doctors running menopause clinics may wish to tailor an individual prescription to your unique needs, and in either of these cases the progestogen tablets may be provided separately to the oestrogen tablets. When this scenario arises, for convenience doctors may recommend that the progestogens are taken for the first 10 to 14 days of each calendar month starting, say, on 1 November or 1 December, which provides you with the advantage that the type and dose of oestrogen and progestogen can be adjusted in the future more easily. Furthermore, since the withdrawal bleed can be expected around the middle of the month any irregular bleeding which occurs, which has not been foreseen can be quickly reported and investigated. On the whole, doctors generally prescribe common brand names of sequential combined HRT and these are listed in Figure 24.

Figure 24

'Sequential Combined'
Oestrogen/Progestogen HRT Tablets

Brand	Oestrogen	Progestogen
Climagest	Oestradiol (1mg, 2mg)	Norethisterone (1mg)
Cycloprogynova	Oestradiol (1mg, 2mg)	Levonorgestrel (0.25mg/0.5mg)
Elleste Duet	Oestradiol (1mg, 2mg)	Norethisterone (1mg)
Femoston 1/10	Oestradiol (1mg)	Dydrogesterone (10mg)
Femoston 2/10	Oestradiol (2mg)	Dydrogesterone (10mg)
Femoston 2/20	Oestradiol(2mg)	Dydrogesterone (20mg)
Premique Cycle	Conjugated oestrogens (0.625mg)	Medroxyprogesterone acetate (10mg)
Prempak C	Conjugated oestrogens (0.625mg, 1.25mg)	Norgestrel (150mcg)
Trisequens	Oestradiol (2mg, 2mg, 1mg) or (4mg, 4mg, 1mg)	Norethisterone (1mg)
Tridestra*	Oestradiol (2mg) acetate	Medroxyprogesterone (20mg)

N.B.   * Tridestra is another type of sequential combined HRT tablet formulation but, unlike the others which produce a monthly bleed, it is designed to produce a 'period' only every three months.

Prescriptions for the above combined HRT preparations incur two prescription charges as more than one hormone is contained in separate tablets. Each preparation is designed to produce a regular monthly bleed.

Finally, if you are more than one year past the menopause (in other words you have not had a period for more than one year), progestogen tablets can be taken every day continuously without a break together with oestrogen, in which case no withdrawal bleeding should occur at all, in an HRT regimen known as 'no bleed HRT' (see Figure 25).

Figure 25

'No bleed HRT' or 'continuous combined HRT'
Designed to prevent 'periods' altogether

Brand	Oestrogen	Progestogen
Climesse	Oestradiol (2mg)	Norethisterone (0.7mg)
Elleste Duet Conti	Oestradiol (2mg)	Norethisterone (1mg)
Kliofem	Oestradiol (2mg)	Norethisterone (1mg)
Kliovance	Oestradiol (1mg)	Norethisterone (0.5mg)
Nuvelle Continuous	Oestradiol (2mg)	Norethisterone (1mg)
Premique	Conjugated oestrogens (0.625mg)	Medroxyprogesterone acetate (5mg)
Femoston Conti	Oestradiol (1mg)	Dydrogesterone (5mg)

N.B.   Prescriptions for the above no-bleed HRT incur only one prescription charge as the two hormones are combined together in a single daily tablet.

Tibolone (brand name Livial) is also designed to prevent periods altogether but is classed as a 'gonado mimetic' rather than a form of HRT. It is taken in a single daily dosage of 2.5mg.

Pros and Cons of HRT Tablets

Although HRT tablets are the most commonly prescribed form of HRT, there are advantages and disadvantages. Certainly they are convenient to take and should any side effects occur they can be quickly reversed simply by omitting to take any further tablets. On the other hand, some people find taking tablets every day difficult to remember and when this happens fluctuations in blood hormone levels will occur, leading to irregular bleeding. Oral HRT also uses high doses of hormones, since they have to be absorbed through the intestine and survive metabolism in the liver before they can act, so these relatively high dosages can lead to an increased possibility of side effects. Nausea, for example, is not uncommonly reported as an occasional side effect of oral HRT although if a tablet is taken with meals or at bedtime the problem may be avoided. Some women appear not to be able to absorb oral oestrogen very well and find that their symptoms are inadequately relieved. For them an alternative type of HRT may be more helpful. Lastly, tablets may also have the disadvantage of being associated with the stigma of 'medication'. Psychologically this may reinforce any negative cultural attitudes towards the menopause, emphasising in the woman's own mind any preconceived ideas she might have that her menopause is a medical illness of some sort.

Skin Patches

HRT skin patches resemble flesh-coloured waterproof sticking plasters in a circular shape. The earliest skin patches consisted of a fairly thick plastic which protected a central fluid bubble containing oestradiol dissolved in alcohol. These were known as 'reservoir' patches. The latest varieties are thinner because instead of possessing a bubble in the middle the hormone is mixed into the adhesive. These so-called 'matrix' patches look better, although younger women may need to use a larger patch or even two. They can also become creased after being worn for a day or two and they can discolour around the edges. Unlike ordinary sticking plasters, however, they are at least less likely to fall off in the shower or bath.

Oestrogen Patches

These patches contain oestradiol which is absorbed from the underside of the patch, through the skin and the subcutaneous fat beneath it, directly into the bloodstream. The oestrogen does not first pass through the intestine, or the liver (unlike tablets), so the required dose can be much lower, which reduces potential side effects. Furthermore, although some of the oestrogen is converted into oestrone, the majority stays as oestradiol. This is beneficial in that blood levels of oestradiol can be monitored to some extent and because the oestrone-oestradiol ratio in the blood mirrors more closely the ratio found naturally in pre-menopausal women. For this reason the effect of HRT patches has been described as being more physiological.

Another benefit is that the hormone contained in the matrix patch is absorbed in a steady trickle over many hours, whereas the hormone absorbed from tablets comes in a single peak.

Depending on the brand, the patches are changed once or twice weekly. It does not matter if another patch has to be used earlier than expected, if a previous one falls off accidentally, because as the new patch is no stronger than the previous one and the hormone is only released in a steady trickle, the overall dose will be the same. The only way to increase the dose, in fact, is to increase the area of skin which is in contact with the patches. This may mean using a larger patch or even more than one patch at a time. Current sizes and doses currently include 25, 40, 50, 75, 80 and 100 microgrammes (mcg). Dose adjustment can occur by wearing two different sizes or even by cutting one patch in half. To give a general idea, if you are around the age of 50 and are in a natural menopause you will often require 50 mcg, whereas if you are younger and lack hormones you may require up to 100 mcg, or even more, and your doctor can advise on this.

For additional help with using the patches patient information leaflets are provided, which recommend placing each patch on a clean, dry, unbroken area of skin anywhere below the waist. The waistband area should be avoided as clothes can rub there, and particularly sensitive skin should be avoided as discomfort can occur when the patch is removed.

To use a patch most effectively, it should be removed from its backing sheet and then stuck on to an area of clean dry skin free from talcum powder, body cream or bath oils. Probably the best site is the upper buttock. The patch should be held firmly against the skin for about ten seconds, and then the edges sealed by finger pressure around the edge. Generally speaking the patches will happily stay on whilst you are taking a bath, showering or swimming. The patches are best removed when you are sunbathing or even using a sun bed.

The original reservoir patches contained alcohol which could irritate some women's skin, and even the more modern matrix patches contain an adhesive which may occasionally bring about an allergy. For this reason it is recommended that the site of application of each patch is changed, and that if you worry about being seen wearing a patch, for example when being romantic with your partner or at a public swimming pool, you can be re-assured that leaving a patch off for several hours before the applying the next is perfectly acceptable. No recurrence of menopausal symptoms would take place in that short time-span. If patches leave any remnants of the adhesive, rubbing this off with baby oil can be effective and most high street pharmacists can advise about special wipes specifically designed for people who, for one reason or another, have to wear bandages on a regular basis and need to remove this adhesive more conveniently. For patches containing oestrogen alone see Figure 26. For oestrogen patches combined with progestogen tablets, see Figure 27.

Oestrogen Progestogen Combination

Patches which contain combinations of these two hormones are available both as double patches, with separate pouches for each hormone, or combined in a single patch. The oestrogen-only patches are used twice weekly for the first two weeks of the cycle followed by the double patches for the last two weeks of the cycle. See Figure 28.

Figure 26

Oestrogen only skin patches and gels

Brand	Oestrogen patches
Dermestril	Oestradiol (25 or 50 or 100 mcg)
Estraderm TTS (transdermal)	Oestradiol (25 or 50 or 100 mcg)
Estraderm MX (matrix patch)	Oestradiol (25 or 50 or 75 or 100 mcg)
Evorel	Oestradiol (25 or 50 or 75 or 100 mcg)
Fematrix	Oestradiol (40 or 80 mcg)
Femseven	Oestradiol (50 or 75 or 100 mcg)
Menorest	Oestradiol (37.5 or 50 or 75 mcg)
Progynova TS	Oestradiol (50 or 100 mcg)

Gels	
Oestrogel	Oestradiol (1.5mg)
Sandrena	Oestradiol (0.5mg or 1mg)

Figure 27

Oestrogen skin patches and progestogen tablets
For sequentially combined HRT designed to produce
monthly 'periods'

Brand	Oestrogen patch	Progestogen tablet
Estrapak	Oestradiol (50mcg)	Norethisterone (1mg)
Evorel-Pak	Oestradiol (50mcg)	Norethisterone (1mg)
Femapak	Oestradiol (40mcg or 80mcg)	Dydrogesterone (10mg)

ectomy you will also need progestogen
vithin the implant.

age is the development of a phenom-
ylaxis. This refers to the experience
unter whereby the time which elapses
on and their menopausal symptoms
r and shorter. Strangely, in this situa-
rn and the oestrogen blood levels are
und to be relatively high, so it appears
unity to the action of oestrogen has
ed that, for some women at least, it is
evel of oestrogen in the body which
of *declining* levels which brings about
s. Despite the fact that women who
s may still have high levels, typical
still occur when these levels begin to
pening the lingering effect of the
e taken into account when a new one
igher and higher levels of oestradiol
loodstream, blood levels should be
the implant is replaced, and lower
e utilised. Finally, when implants are
u have been taking a progestogen
continue to take the progestogen for
e last implant to offset any residual
he womb caused by residual implant

e most popular form of HRT and it
ny years. It has recently been made
now comes in two forms, namely
ng of oestradiol, and Sandrena
Figure 24. When you are in your
e normally prescribed two 2.5mg
hly equates to the same sort of dose

Figure 28

Combined oestrogen and progestogen patches
For sequential combined HRT designed to produce
monthly 'periods'

Brand	Oestrogen patch	Combined patch
Estracombi	Oestradiol (50mcg)	Oestradiol (50mcg + Norethisterone (0.25mg)
Evorel Sequi	Oestradiol (50mcg)	Oestradiol (50mcg + Norethisterone (170mcg)
Nuvelle TS	Oestradiol (80mcg)	Oestradiol (50mcg + Levonorgestrel (20mcg)
Evorel Conti	Oestradiol (50mcg)	Norethisterone acetate (170mcg)

N.B. Prescriptions for all the above incur two prescription charges as more than one hormone is contained in separate patches.

Pros and cons of patches

There are pros and cons to HRT in skin patch form. The advantages include a reduction of side effects compared to when using tablets because a lower dose of hormones is used. Also, the effect of the HRT is more physiological. The disadvantage of patches includes fixed dosages so that adjustment is difficult. The tendency for patches to fall off, particularly in hot humid weather, may also be encountered. Skin sensitivity and irritation may prevent use by some women although different brands are always worth trying.

Implants

Implants, small pellets of hormone, may be inserted into the fatty tissue under the skin and will slowly dissolve over several months. The procedure to insert implants has been practised for over 40 years, and is an easily learned technique suitable for GP surgeries, hospital out-patient clinics and community clinics. You are injected with a local anaesthetic to numb the skin so that it does not hurt and then a small incision is made, usually in the lower abdomen (see Figure 29). The hormone pellet or implant is then inserted through the wound, after which the tiny incision is closed with a steri-strip plaster or sometimes a small stitch.

Implants may consist of oestrogen only, which is generally the case, but may sometimes consist of testosterone if you have sexual problems likely to respond to such treatment. Growing evidence suggests that testosterone may increase libido and sexual responsiveness. Some women find that lowered sex drive responds well enough with oestrogen replacement on its own, but some authorities believe that the addition of testosterone in more severe cases can make a significant difference.

Pros and Cons of HRT Implants

An advantage of hormone implants is that they may be inserted immediately at the time of an operation, such as hysterectomy with removal of both ovaries. Their use also means that you do not have to remember to take tablets or change patches all the time, and implants also provide stable levels of the hormone with minimal hormone fluctuations. Compared to other forms of HRT, the implants produce the highest levels of oestrogen over-all, although these still stay within the normal pre-menopausal range, and they may be specifically used because of these characteristics because higher blood levels of oestradiol are needed, for example in the treatment and prevention of osteoporosis. Implants last on average for up to six months before they need to be replaced.

Disadvantages of implants include the fact that they require both a minor surgical procedure and a doctor who needs to be trained in the technique. A suitably equipped treatment room with sterilised instruments and assistance from a nurse are also required. There is the small but possible risk of a wound infection and, rarely, the implant can spontaneously work itself up to skin level again. Usually, however, the implant is difficult to remove once it has been inserted, which can prove problematical if the implant does not suit any one individual. Of course, if

you have not had a hyste
to oppose the oestrogen

One further disadvant
enon known as tachyph
which some women enco
between each implantat
returning becomes shorte
tion when symptoms ret
measured, they are still fo
as if some kind of immu
occurred. It is now believ
not so much the overall l
is important but the effect
the menopausal symptom
have been given implant
menopausal symptoms ca
fall. To prevent this hap
previous implant should b
is implanted. To prevent h
being absorbed into the b
checked carefully before
doses of implants should be
no longer replaced and y
regime as well, you could
two or more years after th
stimulation of the lining of t
secretion.

Oestrogen Gel

In France oestrogen gel is th
has been in use there for ma
available in the UK too, and
Oestrogel containing 1.5
containing 0.5 or 1mg. See
natural menopause you ar
dollops each day, which roug

Figure 28

**Combined oestrogen and progestogen patches
For sequential combined HRT designed to produce
monthly 'periods'**

Brand	Oestrogen patch	Combined patch
Estracombi	Oestradiol (50mcg)	Oestradiol (50mcg +) Norethisterone (0.25mg)
Evorel Sequi	Oestradiol (50mcg)	Oestradiol (50mcg +) Norethisterone (170mcg)
Nuvelle TS	Oestradiol (80mcg)	Oestradiol (50mcg +) Levonorgestrel (20mcg)
Evorel Conti	Oestradiol (50mcg)	Norethisterone acetate (170mcg)

N.B. Prescriptions for all the above incur two prescription charges as more than one hormone is contained in separate patches.

Pros and cons of patches

There are pros and cons to HRT in skin patch form. The advantages include a reduction of side effects compared to when using tablets because a lower dose of hormones is used. Also, the effect of the HRT is more physiological. The disadvantage of patches includes fixed dosages so that adjustment is difficult. The tendency for patches to fall off, particularly in hot humid weather, may also be encountered. Skin sensitivity and irritation may prevent use by some women although different brands are always worth trying.

Implants

Implants, small pellets of hormone, may be inserted into the fatty tissue under the skin and will slowly dissolve over several months. The procedure to insert implants has been practised for over 40 years, and is an easily learned technique suitable for GP surgeries, hospital out-patient clinics and community clinics. You are injected with a local anaesthetic to numb the skin so that it does not hurt and then a small incision is made, usually in the lower abdomen (see Figure 29). The hormone pellet or implant is then inserted through the wound, after which the tiny incision is closed with a steri-strip plaster or sometimes a small stitch.

Implants may consist of oestrogen only, which is generally the case, but may sometimes consist of testosterone if you have sexual problems likely to respond to such treatment. Growing evidence suggests that testosterone may increase libido and sexual responsiveness. Some women find that lowered sex drive responds well enough with oestrogen replacement on its own, but some authorities believe that the addition of testosterone in more severe cases can make a significant difference.

Pros and Cons of HRT Implants

An advantage of hormone implants is that they may be inserted immediately at the time of an operation, such as hysterectomy with removal of both ovaries. Their use also means that you do not have to remember to take tablets or change patches all the time, and implants also provide stable levels of the hormone with minimal hormone fluctuations. Compared to other forms of HRT, the implants produce the highest levels of oestrogen over-all, although these still stay within the normal pre-menopausal range, and they may be specifically used because of these char-acteristics because higher blood levels of oestradiol are needed, for example in the treatment and prevention of osteoporosis. Implants last on average for up to six months before they need to be replaced.

Disadvantages of implants include the fact that they require both a minor surgical procedure and a doctor who needs to be trained in the technique. A suitably equipped treatment room with sterilised instruments and assistance from a nurse are also required. There is the small but possible risk of a wound infec-tion and, rarely, the implant can spontaneously work itself up to skin level again. Usually, however, the implant is difficult to remove once it has been inserted, which can prove problemati-cal if the implant does not suit any one individual. Of course, if

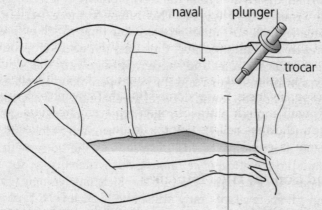

naval   plunger

trocar

at the site of implantation, a small cut is made

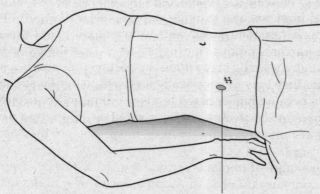

the oestrogen pellet is inserted under the skin into the layer of fat

Figure 29 **The implantation of oestrogen pellets**

you have not had a hysterectomy you will also need progestogen to oppose the oestrogen within the implant.

One further disadvantage is the development of a phenomenon known as tachyphylaxis. This refers to the experience which some women encounter whereby the time which elapses between each implantation and their menopausal symptoms returning becomes shorter and shorter. Strangely, in this situation when symptoms return and the oestrogen blood levels are measured, they are still found to be relatively high, so it appears as if some kind of immunity to the action of oestrogen has occurred. It is now believed that, for some women at least, it is not so much the overall level of oestrogen in the body which is important but the effect of *declining* levels which brings about the menopausal symptoms. Despite the fact that women who have been given implants may still have high levels, typical menopausal symptoms can still occur when these levels begin to fall. To prevent this happening the lingering effect of the previous implant should be taken into account when a new one is implanted. To prevent higher and higher levels of oestradiol being absorbed into the bloodstream, blood levels should be checked carefully before the implant is replaced, and lower doses of implants should be utilised. Finally, when implants are no longer replaced and you have been taking a progestogen regime as well, you could continue to take the progestogen for two or more years after the last implant to offset any residual stimulation of the lining of the womb caused by residual implant secretion.

Oestrogen Gel

In France oestrogen gel is the most popular form of HRT and it has been in use there for many years. It has recently been made available in the UK too, and now comes in two forms, namely Oestrogel containing 1.5mg of oestradiol, and Sandrena containing 0.5 or 1mg. See Figure 24. When you are in your natural menopause you are normally prescribed two 2.5mg dollops each day, which roughly equates to the same sort of dose as you would get from a 50mcg patch, although younger women, who are particularly deficient in hormones, may be advised to use more. The gel is rubbed into the underside of the arms, legs or lower body. It takes a few minutes to dry and the area concerned should not be washed or have any other lotions or creams applied to it for an hour or so. The product packs contain a template in order to illustrate the size of the area to be daubed with the gel so that a fairly accurate dose is applied.

Pros and Cons of HRT Gel

The advantages of oestrogen gel are that it is easy to use, the dose can be easily adjusted and there is no need to mess about with patches or disguise them in public. Also, skin irritation is unlikely. The downside of gel is that it can be inconvenient to wait for the gel to dry before getting dressed, and the other option of applying it before going to bed can be awkward as theoretically the gel can be transferred to a partner's skin from where it can also be absorbed.

Vaginal Oestrogen

Most forms of HRT referred to above are *systemic*, in other words the hormones contained within them are absorbed into the body as a whole and become widely distributed throughout it. Vaginal oestrogen, on the other hand, is only applied locally to the vagina and exerts almost all of its effect in that area. Whereas systemic forms of HRT will have a profound effect on improving vaginal dryness and some urinary problems, vaginal oestrogens generally exert little effect on the rest of the body as so little is absorbed into the bloodstream.

Local oestrogens are available in cream, pessary, vaginal tablet and vaginal ring forms, all of which are relatively simple to use, if somewhat messy. See Figure 30. Products containing natural oestrogens include Vagifem tablets, Ovestin cream, Ortho-Gynest cream and pessaries. Premarin cream contains conjugated equine oestrogens (see page 242), whereas Ortho-dienoestrol cream and Tampovagan pessaries use the synthetic dienoestrol and stilboestrol respectively. It is worth bearing this in mind because the amount of absorption of the hormone into the body can be reduced by using either the vaginal ring or a brand containing natural rather than synthetic oestrogen. Initially cream or pessaries should be used frequently, followed by a reduction fairly soon afterwards as oestrogen absorption occurs more rapidly once the vaginal lining begins to change.

Figure 30

'Local' HRT – Creams, pessaries, vaginal tablets and rings

Oestrogen

Creams	Ortho-Dienoestrol (oestriol cream) 0.01% Ortho-Gynest (oestriol cream) 0.01% Ovestin (oestriol cream) 0.01% Premarin (conjugated oestrogens) 0.625mg per gm
Pessaries	Ortho-Gynest (oestriol) 0.5mg Tampovagan (stilloestrol 0.5mg and lactic acid 5%)
Vaginal tablets	Vagifem (oestradiol) 25mcg
Rings	Estring (oestradiol) 7.5mcg/24hrs

Progestogen

Gel	Crinone (progesterone) 4%
Suppositories (vaginal or rectal)	Cyclogest (progesterone) 200mg/400mg

Pros and Cons of HRT Vaginal Cream

The main advantages of vaginal oestrogen are that there is little risk associated with it and it is very useful for you if you have very few other menopausal symptoms other than a dry vagina, irritation or soreness. It can also be used in addition to systemic HRT formulations if vaginal dryness is responding poorly. Vaginal rings can be inserted at home and will fit you whether you have a cervix or not. Rings are designed to stay in place for three months and to slowly release oestradiol before being renewed. Generally speaking they can be used for up to two years. Disadvantages of vaginal oestrogens are that they can be inconvenient to use in cream or pessary form, although vaginal oestrogen tablets inserted with a special applicator can overcome this difficulty. One major disadvantage is that vaginal creams and other local preparations should not be used indefinitely, especially if you have not had a hysterectomy, because a little absorption of hormone into your body may always occur. Therefore, if local oestrogens are used for more than a few weeks, additional progestogen is sometimes necessary to prevent endometrial stimulation. Premarin cream may in fact be prescribed for long-term use, provided a progestogen is taken for 10 to 14 days each cycle to oppose the action of oestrogen on the womb lining. Finally, it should be remembered that vaginal oestrogen creams should not be used as lubricants for love-making as the hormone can equally well be absorbed by your partner. Leaving a gap of several hours between applying the cream and love-making is recommended.

Tibolone (Livial)

This is an older synthetic drug which acts on oestrogen and progesterone receptors in its own right, but which does not stimulate the lining of the womb. It comes in just one formulation of a 2.5mg daily tablet. Additional cyclical progestogens are unnecessary. It now has a product licence to prevent osteoporosis after the menopause and research studies have suggested that it is certainly effective in this regard; however its ability to prevent heart disease is less clear.

Pros and Cons of Tibolone

The advantage of tibolone is that you can use it if you want to take HRT but do not want to have periods. Another advantage of tibolone is that it is of particular use if you have had endometriosis in the past and your symptoms have returned. As tibolone does not stimulate endometrial tissue it can effectively prevent the re-occurrence of endometriosis, so if you have had your ovaries removed as part of a hysterectomy for this condition it is particularly attractive. Finally, because tibolone also influences receptors which are normally stimulated by testosterone, it is thought to benefit some women whose libido has diminished after the menopause, although the downside is that it can also have possible testosterone-like side effects, such as the growth of unwanted hair and acne. The disadvantage is that if tibolone is used less than 12 months after the last period irregular bleeding can occur, and for this reason it is only recommended for you if you have not had a natural period for at least 12 months. Tibolone is not a contraceptive either.

SERMS

The initials SERMS stand for Selective (o)Estrogen-Receptor Modulators. They are otherwise referred to as 'designer oestrogens' and are currently of interest to research scientists because they may provide a way of circumventing any fears you may have of developing breast cancer whilst taking HRT.

Pros and Cons of SERMS

They are different to the varieties of oestrogen usually used in conventional HRT and, as their name suggests, they work selectively. They work, in fact, in a similar way to Tamoxifen, a standard drug used in the treatment of breast cancer. This blocks the effect of your own oestrogen on breast tissue whilst simultaneously exerting oestrogen-like effects on other parts of the body such as the bones, for example. In other words, these oestrogen receptor modulators are selective because they block some oestrogen receptors whilst stimulating others. In the development stages of these drugs it was therefore hoped that they might be able to increase the level of protection to you (when you are post-menopausal) against osteoporosis, whilst reducing any possible risk of breast cancer at the same time. The first product in this family of medications is now available and is on prescription in Britain under the name of raloxifene (Evista). Although raloxifene has a product licence for the prevention of vertebral osteoporosis in post-menopausal women, it is not however effective in relieving hot flushes and other short-term symptoms of the menopause, which makes it less attractive as a form of hormone therapy anyway. It may be that in years to come further drugs in the SERM family will become available which are so selective that they do everything you might dream a drug could do for you when you are post-menopausal, without causing any problems in return.

Decisions, Decisions

Before making a choice about which of the various different types of HRT you should take it is worth reconsidering their various advantages and disadvantages. These are summarised in Figure 31. Recent forms of HRT have been able to offer additional benefits for some women. Long cycle HRT, for example (Tridestra, Figure 24), means that you take oestrogens every day as usual but only take the progestogen course every three months. This means that you only have four withdrawal bleeds every year. The downside here is that a relatively high dose of progestogen is required, which can occasionally bring about certain side effects as well as causing prolonged or heavy bleeding.

Another option is to prevent withdrawal bleeds altogether by

Figure 31

Advantages and disadvantages of the different forms of HRT

Advantages	Disadvantages
Tablets: Easy to take Easily reversible Cheap	Unnatural delivery of hormone Must be taken daily

Patches:
Convenient
Easy to use
More natural delivery
  of hormone
Easily reversible
	Can irritate the skin
	Can become detached
	More expensive than tablets
	Must be changed once or twice
	  a week

Implants:
100 per cent compliance
More natural delivery
  of hormones
Prolonged effect
  (4–6 months)
Cheap
	Needs a small surgical procedure
	Can cause unnaturally high
	  levels of hormones
	Not easily reversible
	Progestogens need to be continued
	  for several months after final implant

Gel: Easy to use More natural delivery of hormone	Must cover correct amount of skin More expensive than tablets

**Vaginal creams
  and tablets:**
Greater effect if vaginal
  problems are the only
  symptoms
Easily reversible
	Some is absorbed into the bloodstream
	Long-term use needs progestogen
	treatment
	Messy (tablets less so)

Tibolone: No withdrawal bleeds	Only for post-menopausal women Side effect of occasional irregular bleeding Expensive

using a combination of oestrogen and progestogen continuously (Figure 25). This prevents any proliferation of the lining of the womb, which means that any withdrawal bleed becomes unnecessary. Some unpredictable bleeding may occur in the first few months but this usually settles within the first year, and is much less likely to arise when it is used by women who have been post-menopausal for at least a year before they start this form of HRT. If you have been taking cyclical HRT and wish to change to this no-bleed regimen you should wait until the end of a withdrawal bleed before starting on the new tablets. In other words you should take the first few tablets of the next pack of your old cyclical HRT before discontinuing them and starting the new regimen. This is to make sure the lining of the womb will be thin to begin with, to prevent any chances of further bleeding.

By and large the types of HRT regimes used by most women who have not had a hysterectomy fall into the categories shown in Figure 30. Never forget that all women have different experiences of the menopause and require any prescription of HRT to be tailored to their individual needs. Because their response to HRT is also individually unpredictable, it may be necessary to alter the dose or the formulation of the HRT in the first few months after starting therapy. It is logical that if you are having severe symptoms of the menopause you may require a higher dose of oestrogen than if your symptoms are only mild or moderate. When symptoms such as hot flushes and night sweats are not satisfactorily relieved, the dose of oestrogen needs to be adjusted upwards. On the other hand, if side effects of oestrogen are troublesome then the dose may need to be altered downwards. There is, however, a minimum daily dose of oestrogen which is required to protect against bone loss, and in the various preparations available these are 0.625mg of conjugated oestrogens in daily tablets; 2mg of oestradiol in daily tablets; 40 to 50mcg of oestradiol in once or twice weekly patches; 1.5mg of oestradiol in two daily doses of gel; and 50mg of oestradiol in a six monthly implant. Similarly, it is important to obtain the recommended dose of progestogen to eradicate any risk of endometrial cancer. The duration of therapy should be for twelve days in each month but the dose again depends on the type of progestogen used. For these requirements it is 0.7 to 2.5mg of norethisterone; 150mcg of levon-orgestrel; 10 to 20mg of dydrogesterone; 5 to 10mg of medroxyprogesterone acetate; or 200 to 400mg micronised progesterone.

HRT is still most commonly prescribed for the short-term symptoms of the menopause and therefore it is most commonly used at the average age when the menopause occurs and in the years leading up to it, say in the late forties and early fifties. But it is never too late to start HRT at any age, as the risk of osteoporosis and heart disease would still be diminished as you become older. Since osteoporosis begins before the menopause, however, and since the rate of bone mineral density loss accelerates markedly immediately after the menopause, the earlier hormone replacement therapy is started the better. Should you want to start HRT prior to the menopause proper, and you still have monthly bleeding, it may be necessary to make alterations to the timing of the progestogen in order to prevent irregular bleeding.

When Should You Start HRT and How Long Can You Continue With It?

Whilst many women come off their therapy within two to three years of the menopause and notice no recurrence of their hot flushes and night sweats, others continue to take it for as long as five years and when they discontinue treatment still experience these kind of symptoms, although they tend to be less frequent and severe after this time. However, in order to protect against osteoporosis and heart disease in the future, taking HRT for at least five years and probably up to 10 or 15 years is recommended. Provided you are happy taking HRT, provided you feel well and it has no side effects, you can continue to take the treatment as long as you wish. Many women have successfully taken HRT for 20 to 30 years.

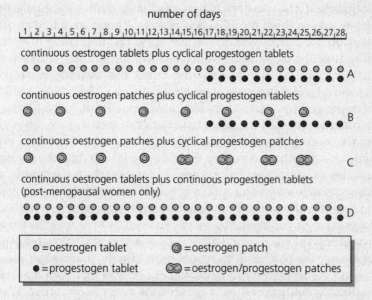

number of days

continuous oestrogen tablets plus cyclical progestogen tablets — A

continuous oestrogen patches plus cyclical progestogen tablets — B

continuous oestrogen patches plus cyclical progestogen patches — C

continuous oestrogen tablets plus continuous progestogen tablets (post-menopausal women only) — D

○ = oestrogen tablet   ◎ = oestrogen patch
● = progestogen tablet   ◎◎ = oestrogen/progestogen patches

A oestrogen tablets are taken daily plus progestogen tablets for 10 to 14 days monthly

B oestrogen patches are applied once or twice weekly plus progestogen tablets are taken for 10 to 14 days monthly

C oestrogen patches are applied twice weekly for two weeks, plus double patches of progestogen combined with oestrogen tablets are applied twice weekly for the other two weeks of the month

D continuous oestrogen tablets plus continuous progestogen tablets for women who have been post-menopausal for the last twelve months

Figure 32 **HRT regimens for women who have not had a hysterectomy**

Stopping HRT

Bearing in mind that HRT works by replacing hormones which have become deficient after the menopause, stopping HRT abruptly can potentially lead to a recurrence of symptoms. To stop this happening, when you wish to discontinue your HRT you should tail the dose down gradually over a timescale of about two to three months. It is always a good idea to consult your doctor before you do this anyway. The first thing to do is to reduce the dose of oestrogen, whilst continuing to take the progestogen at the usual time until the oestrogen stops completely. For example, if you are using a 1.25mg daily tablet of oestrogen you can reduce to a tablet containing just 0.625mg, in other words half the dose. Later you can increase the interval between each dose, for example you can take the tablet on alternate days then on every third day or fourth day. If you use patches you can again use a lower dose patch, for example a 25mcg patch instead of a 50mcg patch and then later you can leave extra days free between replacing each patch. Another alternative, if you are using matrix patches, is to reduce the dose by cutting the patch into half or into quarters whilst continuing to replace the patches at the usual time. Finally, if you have been relying on oestrogen implants you can ensure that each dose of implant is reduced when it is replaced every six months. You should, however, then continue to take regular courses of progestogen until there is no further bleeding, which may take up to two or three years.

CHAPTER 16

DECISIONS – IS HRT FOR YOU?

With so many conflicting opinions about the pros and cons of hormone replacement therapy, it can be very difficult for anybody to decide whether or not they should take it. Most medical information for women is gained from newspaper articles, magazine features and broadcasting, but much of this information is inaccurate, out of date, commercially orientated or simply erroneous. Scare stories about HRT abound. Then again, not every woman needs HRT, many do not wish to take it, others for medical reasons simply should not take it, and many are disuaded from trying it because of the perceived side effects and risks. On top of all this, female celebrities from stage and screen are often heard waxing lyrical about the wonders of HRT and how it has revolutionised their lives, whereas vociferous minority groups campaign tirelessly about the dangers of HRT, claiming that the pharmaceutical industry is taking advantage of vulnerable women purely to line their own pockets.

What is the truth? How can you possibly come to a sensible conclusion in light of all this? Some menopausal women seem happy and relieved to leave all decision-making to their own doctor. At a time when they may feel anxious, uncertain and possibly even confused about the way ahead, the sympathetic advice from a trusted doctor may offer the very stability for which they crave. Others amongst you will feel very strongly that you want to play a vital role in the decision-making process and seek to accumulate as much background information as is humanly possible. Some women clearly remain unimpressed by their family doctor's general lack of knowledge about HRT, a fact which many good GPs are willing to admit to in the light of frequent and constant changes in HRT types and formulations.

Certain doctors might acquiesce in suggestions made by patients, which may or may not be appropriate; some doctors are willing to refer to local hospital gynaecology clinics, whereas others are not. To some extent menopausal health care has become something of a lottery. In this chapter I am going to offer a logical approach to coming to a decision about whether or not to take HRT, and attempt to end the confusion.

Women are Individuals

No two women will experience identical symptoms of the menopause. There are so many different types of physical and psychological symptoms associated with the change, and so many different attitudes towards it, that each of you must be looked upon as a unique individual. It is only by taking an holistic approach to helping you through the menopause that a satisfactory outcome can be attained. Some will have been baffled by conflicting statistics with which they have come into contact, and some, because of their own life experience, will have particular fears about factors such as breast cancer or heart disease. Some of you, in consultation with your doctor, will simply want advice about how to alleviate symptoms associated with the menopause, and others will be interested in longer-term therapy which benefits their heart and keeps their bones strong.

Strangely, this more enlightened attitude to long-term therapy is a fairly recent one. Most women are, in fact, much more likely to die from heart disease than from breast cancer and yet, when considering whether to take HRT, most women immediately consider the breast cancer implications. The number one killer of women in the UK overall is coronary heart disease, claiming hundreds of thousands of lives every year. In comparison, breast cancer is responsible for far fewer deaths. It is true to say that among women younger than 75, there are actually three times as many deaths from heart disease as there are from breast cancer. In addition, one in three women over the age of 50 are likely to go on to develop an osteoporotic fracture, with all the disability and discomfort that that may bring. Whilst these statistics describe the experiences of entire populations, they do not tell us much about you as an individual. This is because the risks for developing coronary heart disease, breast cancer and osteoporosis vary considerably from one individual to another, depending upon personal characteristics, family history and lifestyle. So whilst the average risk in a lifetime for developing breast cancer might be one in 12, for an individual woman it could be one in 50 or one in two, depending on her unique situation.

It is your personal characteristics which will determine whether HRT will benefit you or not and, furthermore, any decision committing you to taking HRT long term should be made in the light of your personal medical history and situation because unlike the statistical 'mean', you yourself cannot be regarded as 'average'.

HRT and Prolonged Life Expectancy

Taking HRT can make a huge difference to your life. This is true not only in terms of controlling inconvenient and sometimes disabling short-term symptoms of the menopause, but HRT can actually prolong life expectancy by up to three years in certain individuals. For example, if you are a 50-year-old lady who smokes, who has high blood pressure and an elevated cholesterol level in your blood, you can expect to live around three years longer by taking HRT. Conversely, if you do not smoke and have normal blood pressure and low cholesterol, but your mother and sister had breast cancer, you might well live longer by *not* taking HRT. Looking at the hypothetical concept of an 'average' woman, it is, however, true to say that such a woman can expect to live about six months longer with HRT. But, as I say, all women should be treated as unique, individuals. A very rough idea about whether HRT might prolong *your* life expectancy, as well as improve the quality of *your* life, can be gained by completing the following life expectancy rapid assessment chart.

Rapid Assessment Chart

If you are a woman of under 60 years of age and in general good health, you, like everybody else, may award yourself a four-month gain in life expectancy. This is accounted for in the top line of the chart (see page 309). Add or subtract the number of months according to the answers to each listed question on the chart. This number will tell you the number of months gained or lost by taking HRT. Add up the total at the bottom of the chart.

Jackie and Jane have completed their own assessments in the two right-hand columns, and you can see how they have completed the chart according to their own personal circumstances by reading about their details below.

Now fill in the assessment chart yourself, in the same way, and discover whether HRT is likely to prolong your own life expectancy or not.

Looking at Jackie's example, she is in good general health so she starts with an extra four months of life expectancy. Nobody in her family has suffered from breast cancer nor has Jackie herself had any benign or malignant breast lumps diagnosed. Her LDL cholesterol levels, however, when measured at a Well Woman Clinic proved to be moderately raised so she scores an extra eight months, as HRT is known to be helpful in reducing 'bad' cholesterol levels and protecting against heart disease. Her blood pressure is consistently measured by her doctor at 150/90 (the higher reading being known as the 'systolic' reading) and because it is above average, Jackie can expect an extra two months of life expectancy as HRT is known to relax blood vessels and prevent hardening of the arteries which may cause strokes and heart disease in the future. Jackie can also add two months as her mother fell and fractured her hip at the age of 73, suggesting a family history of osteoporosis which HRT again helps to protect against.

Jackie's score when totted up is therefore +16 months which translates as meaning that she can expect to live a healthy 16 months longer by taking HRT now than if she did not.

Jane's score, on the other hand, is zero as her family history of

Risk Factor	Jackie's score	Jane's score	Your score
You are in good general health (start with 4 months)	+ 4	+ 4	+ 4
You have one close relative with breast cancer – 2 months You have two close relatives with breast cancer – 6 months		– 2	
You have had one previous benign breast lump – 1 month You have had two previous benign breast lumps – 2 months		– 2	
Your level of LDL (bad cholesterol) is Average + 3 months Your level of LDL (bad cholesterol) is Slightly raised + 6 months Your level of LDL (bad cholesterol) is Moderately raised + 8 months Your level of LDL (bad cholesterol) is Significantly raised + 11 months	+8		
Your systolic blood pressure (the higher of the two figures, e.g. 140/80) is between 135 and 144 + 1 month is between 145 and 154 + 2 months is between 155 and 164 + 3 months is over 164 + 4 months	+ 2		
You have a family history of hip fracture or a bone mineral density of 1 or more standard deviations below average (as measured by a DXA scan, see page 146) + 2 months	+ 2		
Estimated gain or loss of life expectancy	+ 16 months	0 months	

breast cancer counts against her (as HRT *may* influence breast cancer unfavourably) and because she has had two benign breast lumps diagnosed herself. The four months subtracted from her initial start-out score of four months brings her back to zero, and in the absence of any risk factors for osteoporosis and heart disease this is how her score stays. In her situation then, Jane would be no better off taking HRT than not taking it as far as life expectancy goes.

The rapid assessment chart is only a rough guide to life expectancy assessment, and should not be relied upon too closely. But it does at least provide some idea of the various factors which might help you come to a decision about how useful HRT might or might not be in prolonging your life.

The above chart is calculated for women under the age of 60. If you are 60 or older, the number you have just calculated needs to be adjusted according to your age. For each five years of age over 60, you should reduce your life expectancy if taking HRT by one month. For example, if Jackie in the above chart were 70, her estimated gained life expectancy would be +14 months rather than +16 months. This, again, is a calculation based on the fact that the woman concerned is in general good health and not suffering from any chronic disorder.

HRT May Be Taken for Different Reasons

It never occurs to many women that taking HRT might extend their life expectancy and many women still only use it for short-lived troublesome symptoms of the menopause. HRT used in this situation can be very effective and many women find that when they discontinue their HRT after two to three years their symptoms either do not return or if they do are extremely mild and entirely bearable. Others notice side effects in the first few weeks of therapy for one reason or another, and up to 30 per cent of women prescribed HRT discontinue treatment within the first three or four months. A significant proportion of women feel so much better and healthier, however, on HRT that after five years they feel determined to continue with their treatment, confident in the knowledge that they have already had substantial benefits and can look forward to the less obvious but nevertheless more important ones which include long-term protection against osteoporosis and heart disease.

Long-Term Post-Menopausal Risks

The three greatest long-term health risks you run post-menopausally are heart disease, osteoporosis and breast cancer – in that order. At least, this is the case for the average women amongst you. However, you as an individual may be at higher risk of any one of these three disorders because of certain factors. For example, if you are at higher risk of developing heart disease, you can expect to obtain greater benefit from taking HRT. So if the blood pressure is raised, if cholesterol levels are high, if you are diabetic, if you smoke cigarettes, if you have a strong family history of heart disease, and if you take very little physical exercise, you might be well advised to consider taking HRT because it will provide you with extra protection.

Similarly, if you are at higher risk of osteoporosis because of particular factors then again you might be well advised to consider HRT to offer such extra protection. If there is a strong family history of osteoporosis, if you take little exercise, if you are tall and thin, if your bone mineral density is less than normal, if you smoke and drink, and if your diet is low in calcium, you might do very well to think about the additional advantages of taking HRT.

Conversely, you might be at greater risk than average for developing breast cancer. Risk factors for breast cancer include a strong family history of breast cancer, such as having a mother, sister, half-sister or daughter who has developed breast cancer themselves. Also, previous non-cancerous breast lumps requiring biopsies make the risk of breast cancer slightly higher. Starting periods at an early age (say, younger than 14) and having a first child later in life (say, 30 years or older) also increases the risk. Most significantly, if you are known to carry certain breast cancer genes, such as the BRCA1 and BRCA2 genes, you will certainly be at greater risk of developing breast cancer and therefore HRT would not be appropriate. In the light of current scientific knowledge you should avoid HRT as the oestrogen component within it could feasibly stimulate breast cancer cells and detrimentally affect medical outcome.

Attitudes Towards HRT

Some of you may have problems deciding whether to take HRT, not because of medical considerations but because of feelings and attitudes. Some of you need to consider whether HRT is *natural* or not. You may be concerned about whether HRT is *necessary* or not. You may want to explore alternatives, and you might simply regard 'steroids' generally as being unwholesome and potentially dangerous. If you belong to this last group, you should be reassured by the fact that steroids are a huge group of naturally occurring substances which govern many life-giving processes within the body, and that steroid therapy, when used appropriately, has saved many millions of lives. A small number of women cannot come to terms with the knowledge that some forms of HRT are derived from pregnant mares' urine, and they have ethical difficulties with that (see page 242).

All of these conceptual uncertainties, together with attitudes towards minor side effects should they arise in the first few weeks of therapy, are matters on which the family doctor is very well placed to advise, both before treatment is even considered and during the initial frequent check-ups thereafter. A thorough, caring and sympathetic doctor, whether male or female, can provide much of the essential information to help you make up your mind about HRT. He or she can explode many of the myths which still abound, and which still dreadfully confuse some women. He or she can explain how HRT works, what are the pros and cons, what alternatives are available and what you can expect from treatment. The family doctor should thoroughly assess you holistically as an individual and in your own unique situation. He or she should discuss dietary measures, exercise and other lifestyle factors, and certainly encourage you to avail yourself of medical screening at this important time in your life. Your GP should also carry out base line checks (see page 277) before HRT is begun and make arrangements to reassess you at three months, six months and then at least annually thereafter.

The Decision is Yours

Post-menopausal hormone therapy is a complex intervention that produces some positive and some adverse health effects. In the vast majority of cases the benefits of therapy will outweigh the risks. This conclusion is largely based on the cardiovascular benefits of hormone therapy, along with protection against osteoporosis. Any small increase in the risk of breast cancer is more than balanced out by these advantages. Doctors call such conclusions 'decision analyses', which are confirmed by observational studies of mortality in women who use hormones versus women who do not.

These studies report a 30–50 per cent reduction in mortality in women who use HRT compared to those who do not. One decision analysis even concluded that if you have at least one risk factor for coronary heart disease (even if you have a first-degree relative with breast cancer) you could still expect a gain in life expectancy from using hormone therapy.

At the end of the day, the value that each of you individually places on the various health outcomes associated with HRT differs. Any decision as to whether or not to use HRT must be made jointly by you and your doctor, who should take into account all known and possible benefits and risks in the light of your own medical history and current state of health as well as, of course, most important of all, your own personal point of view.

PART FIVE

CHAPTER 17

COMMON QUESTIONS, STRAIGHTFORWARD ANSWERS

Hopefully, this book will have already answered many of your questions about the menopause, but others will always crop up. The following are the most common questions that I encounter on a day-to-day basis.

Q. *My poor old mother lost about 6 inches in height in the last 20 years of her life, and although she suffered a lot of pain, I don't think she was ever offered any treatment. I understand osteoporosis can run in families. Is there anything I can do at this stage? I'm now 52 and want to stop the same thing happening to me.*

A. A lot depends on your natural size, shape and lifestyle, whether you take plenty of weight-bearing exercise, and enjoy a healthy diet containing plenty of calcium and vitamin D, for example. These factors will reduce any future risk. If you are tall and thin rather than short and well covered this will tend to increase your risk, as the absence of fat stores reduces the amount of oestrogen stored within your body. Oestrogen, remember, is necessary to maintain bone mineral density. Also, if you smoke or drink a lot of alcohol, this tends to interfere with the action of calcium in keeping your bones strong. But at 52 you will have gone through or will be going through the menopause, and because your oestrogen levels will be falling, the best preventative treatment for you is to replace that missing oestrogen by using hormone replacement therapy. This should be taken for at least five years, but preferably much longer to give maximum benefit to the bones. If, after discussing HRT with your doctor, you decide between you that it is not appropriate in your case, then there are alternatives which are non-hormonal, such as the so-called biphosphonate group of drugs which are available on prescription. Talk to your doctor also about the possibility of having a DXA scan to assess the density of your bones if you are in a high risk group.

Q. Now I have gone through the menopause, one of the things I worry about most is breast cancer. We hear so much about it in the media but I simply don't feel confident about examining my own breasts as I've never been trained to do this, and how could I possibly be as thorough and effective as a trained doctor?

A. Strange though it may seem, you probably are the most appropriate person to be examining your own breasts for unusual lumps or other changes. Yes, your doctor can examine your breasts from time to time but he or she does not have the benefit of knowing what your breasts are like all the time. You do. Research has confirmed that personal breast awareness is actually more likely to detect an early lump than opportunistic screening carried out by trained doctors in clinics, hospitals or family practices. It is good practice to ask your doctor or practice nurse to check your breasts on the first occasion and to teach you what you are feeling for. Then practise on yourself every one or two months so you get to know what is normal for you as an individual. That way, if you carry out the same examination each time, you are very likely to notice any changes very easily. If anything at all worries you, whether it is a change in the size or shape of the breast, puckering of the skin, inversion or discharge from a nipple, discomfort or the presence of a lump, then do not hesitate to consult your doctor. In nine out of ten cases, a breast lump will not be malignant, but if there is a lump present, the earlier investigations are carried out, the earlier the detection of a possible cancer can occur. For more detailed instructions on how to examine your breasts, see page 172.

Q. Now I have all the information I need about the menopause and HRT, I'm wondering who I should see and where I should go to obtain the correct prescription. Should I simply go to my family doctor or a specialist clinic, and is there anything I should do immediately before and in the first few months after my HRT is started?

A. It would seem the simplest and most convenient thing to see your own GP first as you might be lucky and find he or she has a special interest in gynaecology, the menopause and HRT. However, there are many GPs who will be honest with you and admit that they are almost as bewildered as you are about the various different forms of HRT now available. If this is the situation you are entitled to ask to be referred to the local hospital clinic, and your doctor can write a letter on your behalf setting out your medical history. You could also call an organisation such as the Amarant Trust (see Useful Addresses) who can advise over the phone or arrange a specialist appointment for you. Your personal and family history needs to be taken into consideration, and then you should have a general check-up which will include a blood test, a urine test, height and weight checks, blood pressure tests, breast examination, internal examination and a cervical smear. If you are over 50 you are likely to be encouraged to join the NHS national mammography screening campaign, although it is not essential that you have a mammogram before HRT is started. Ideally, you should be reviewed three months after beginning your HRT, when you can report how your symptoms have responded and whether or not there are any side effects. If all is well you will probably be reviewed again in six months, and thereafter at annual intervals. If any symptoms occur in the meantime, of course, a doctor's appointment should be made in the usual way, for reassurance if nothing else.

Q. I have the most awful night sweats where I have to throw the covers off my soaking body, rush over to the window and throw it open even in the middle of winter. This, of course, drives my husband mad, but it is truly distressing and I'm getting very little sleep. I also have terrible hot flushes during the day and I am therefore thinking of starting HRT. However, there is a strong family history of breast cancer as both of my sisters are currently being treated for breast cancer. In view of this would HRT be safe for me to take?

A. Since you have two sisters who have had breast cancer, it would be logical for you to ask your doctor about whether you can be genetically tested to see if you carry the gene which would make breast cancer more likely in your own case. If so, current medical opinion would recommend that you avoid HRT to reduce any future risks. There are, however, good alternatives for the control of hot flushes and night sweats when simple self-help measures prove unsatisfactory (see Chapter 12). I'm sure you have already taken measures to wear only the very coolest nightwear, ideally made from pure cotton, and have ventilated your bedroom as well as possible. Avoiding hot spicy foods and hot drinks is also very worth while. Recent research on phyto-estrogens, the oestrogens derived from plant material, has shown that increasing your dietary intake of isoflavones can have quite a dramatic effect on hot flushes and night sweats, and this is quite feasible to achieve. There is no current evidence that phytoestrogens promote breast cancer, but much to suggest they may very well possess a significant cancer protective effect instead. Using more soya based products and enjoying more legumes, in addition to special isoflavone supplements from health shops will probably improve your symptoms by up to 50 per cent. Alternatively, there are non-hormonal preparations such as clonidine which you might like to try on prescription.

Q. I went through a fairly straightforward menopause at 47 and apart from a few months of irregular bleeding, I had no great problems. There is, however, in my family a history of heart disease and now that I am 61, I wondered if HRT would be a good idea as I have recently learnt that it can protect the heart and increase life expectancy. A return to having periods, however, at my age would be quite unsatisfactory. Is there any way round this?

A. I'm delighted to be able to tell you that 'bleed free' HRT is now available, which means you can derive all the benefits of HRT without having any periods. With these formulations you take progestogen and oestrogen together on a daily basis without any monthly break. It is completely safe, and as you say, it offers good protection against heart disease, especially in someone who has a family history. The fact that it also protects against brittle bone disease is simply a bonus.

Q. I'm only 42 but I'm having more frequent periods some of which are abnormally heavy. How do I know if this is a symptom of early menopause or a symptom of something more sinister?

A. It is quite possible that the change in the pattern of your periods is due to a relatively early menopause, although you do not mention any other menopausal symptoms and there are, of course, other possibilities. The only way to sort this out is to have some simple investigations which will include a blood test, to measure hormone levels, as well as an internal examination and a cervical smear to rule out any other obvious problems. If there is no other abnormality yet the hormone levels are strongly suggestive of the menopause, there are a number of options available to you which could control your irregular periods and treat any other menopausal symptoms which may soon arise. At your relatively young age you would not want the inconvenience of very frequent periods going on for too long, and medical or possibly even surgical choices are open to you. HRT is certainly a possibility which would not only ease any short-term symptoms of the menopause but protect you long term from osteoporosis and heart disease too.

Q. I started treatment with HRT when I went through the menopause at the age of 49. I have been having a monthly bleed ever since then, but a friend of mine is taking something she calls period-free HRT and I wondered if I can switch to this myself and how would I go about it?

A. Your doctor can decide if period-free or 'no bleed' HRT is suitable for you, and if you are prescribed it, switching from a monthly bleed HRT to a period-free HRT is relatively simple. All you need to do is to wait until your period begins and then stop taking your current HRT. Then, when your period finishes you can start taking your new period-free HRT as instructed by your doctor.

Q. If I have a hysterectomy will I put on a lot of weight afterwards?

A. Having a hysterectomy in itself will not make you gain weight, but anybody who has a major operation and is relatively less active during a fairly extended recovery period is likely to gain a few extra pounds. You might also look as if you have gained a little weight as there will be a fullness in the lower abdomen as a result of the abdominal muscles being stretched and losing some of their tone in the first few weeks after the operation. By sticking to a low fat diet and gradually increasing the amount of regular aerobic-type exercise you take, with some abdominal crunch exercises thrown in, you should soon be able to lose that weight and pull in the stomach. Before you leave hospital the physiotherapist can provide you with an exercise plan to get you started.

Q. *I've been offered a hysterectomy for very heavy and irregular bleeding but I must say I am anxious that I will feel somehow less of a woman and be less romantically inclined towards my husband thereafter. Can you reassure me?*

A. There is no reason whatsoever why having a hysterectomy should affect your sex life in the future. As the well-known saying goes, in this operation you lose the nursery, but you still have the playpen. And because you do not have to worry any more about unpredictable vaginal bleeding, abdominal bloating or discomfort, many women find that their sex life actually improves. In terms of your sexuality and femininity, these should remain unaffected provided, of course, that you have been contributing to the decision-making process in your treatment and that you have embarked upon the hysterectomy fully informed and confident about the pros and cons. If you have a positive mental attitude to the operation it is much more likely to be a resounding success. Let me further reassure you that losing the uterus is highly unlikely to reduce sexual arousal or fulfilment. If, however, there were relationship or sexual difficulties within the relationship before a hysterectomy, the operation itself will not of course remedy these. Anatomically and physiologically you would still be fine, but in this situation some psycho-sexual counselling would be required.

Q. *When can I drive again after a hysterectomy?*

A. There is no hard and fast rule about when you can drive after this operation, and a lot depends on whether the womb was removed through the abdominal or vaginal route. The abdominal operation generally takes longer to recover from, the average being three to four weeks. Once some regular exercises have begun and the wound is comfortable, much depends on how you feel when you are sitting in a chair with your knees tucked up towards your chest. Generally speaking most women will be driving after about a month.

Q. I've been booked in for a hysterectomy and have been told I can expect the operation in about two to three months time. I was asked whether I would prefer a vaginal or an abdominal hysterectomy, but I really have no idea which is best. What is the main difference?

A. Whilst vaginal hysterectomy as an operation is generally easier to perform and safer to have performed than the abdominal variety, not everybody is suitable for this type of procedure. It is excellent where there is a degree of prolapse of the womb, and in women who have had children and have some weakness of the pelvic floor muscles. Other women, however, who might have large fibroids in their womb or a condition known as endometriosis will almost certainly be recommended to have an abdominal hysterectomy. Much obviously depends on the individual. Generally speaking, the gynaecologist will have a personal preference for the type of operation you are offered, and since it is likely that he or she will be the one carrying out the procedure, there is a certain logic in going along with that, unless you have particular reasons for not doing so.

Q. What causes bladder control problems?

A. Amongst some of the other possible causes, weak pelvic floor muscles, which support the bladder outlet, may have been stretched and weakened during childbirth. The menopause itself can cause vaginal dryness and increase the frequency of bladder infections too. Being overweight puts an added strain on the pelvic floor muscles, and certain drugs, constipation or even anxiety can lead to difficulties with bladder control. Thankfully, the most common forms of bladder weakness may be prevented by performing pelvic floor exercises on a regular basis. Referral to a local continence or physiotherapy clinic can start the ball rolling, and medical and surgical options are available in more severe cases.

Q. How does oestrogen help in preventing heart disease?

A. Many research studies have shown the benefits of oestrogen in the reduction of cardiovascular disease. After 10 years of treatment the reduction in risk of heart disease may be as high as 60 per cent. This may be due to the effect of oestrogens reversing the increase in total blood cholesterol, or in reversing the decrease in so-called 'good cholesterol' (HDL) which is associated with the menopause. By reversing the process, which otherwise leads to hardening of the arteries, the coronary arteries which supply the heart muscle with oxygen and other nutrients do not get clogged and the risk of heart attacks and angina is therefore reduced.

Q. Why are horses used in the production of some forms of HRT?

A. Mares are one of the few mammals which produce high levels of oestrogens during pregnancy which are very similar indeed to those produced by women. Several appear to be unique to pregnant mares, making them the only suitable source of natural conjugated oestrogen. These oestrogens contain a unique complex of ten biologically active components, all derived from pregnant mares' urine, which is then put through complex processes involving more than 125 stages (see page 242 for more detail). All other oestrogens are, to a varying degree, manufactured synthetically from chemicals and contain only one, two or three oestrogens.

Q. Is there an HRT treatment made from yams? I think I read about one which claims it can improve my sex life.

A. Perhaps the article you are referring to was titled, 'Wham, bam, thank you Yam', published in *Women and Extra*. There are natural progesterone creams, such as Progest, which are derived from wild yam extract and recommended by some nutritionists as an acceptable alternative to HRT. However, they remain unlicensed products at the current time as there are no randomised controlled trials that show any clear benefits. Whilst anecdotal evidence suggests that these might be useful for the control of hot flushes, no studies have shown it can reduce the risk of osteoporosis or heart disease. Furthermore, the long-term safety of such products and their ability to get into the bloodstream in sufficient doses to be effective have never been demonstrated. At present the only way to obtain such products is on private prescription sent to special pharmaceutical outlets or on the Internet. Talking to your doctor first is therefore highly recommended.

Q. My periods have become erratic over the past few months, but I can honestly say that apart from that I am not suffering from any physical symptoms of the menopause. I do, however, sometimes feel that I am losing my mind as I find it hard to concentrate, I often become tearful, I simply cannot sleep well at night and have become irritable and moody. Not like me at all! Is this a recognised part of the menopause and what on earth can I do to escape from these symptoms?

A. These symptoms could very well be related to your menopause as some women experience psychological symptoms rather than physical ones. However, there are of course other possibilities, including depression, which can occur at any time of life including the menopause. Possibly the two are interrelated and treatment should be tailored to suit you as an individual. I think it would be appropriate for you to have your hormone levels measured to confirm that you are indeed menopausal, and then you need to be fully assessed in an extended appointment with your doctor to see whether your symptoms are predominantly menopausal or due to depression. At that stage a decision can be made about the most appropriate treatment for you, which should be reviewed on a regular basis, perhaps every fortnight for a few weeks, to monitor progress. Both depression and the menopause are eminently treatable, and I have no doubt you will soon be back in control of your life.

CHAPTER 18

USEFUL ADDRESSES

The Amarant Trust
Sycamore House
5 Sycamore Street
London EC1Y 0SR

British Acupuncture Council
Park House
206-208 Latimer Road
London W10 6RE

British Association for
Counselling
1 Regent Place
Rugby
Warwickshire CV21 2PJ

British Chiropractic Association
17 Blagrave Street
Reading
Berkshire RG1 1QB

British Heart Foundation
14 Fitzhardinge Street
London W1H 4DH

British Massage Therapy Council
3 Woodhouse Cliff
Headingley
Leeds
West Yorkshire LS6 2Hf

British School of Osteopathy
275 Borough High Street
London SE1 1JE

Cancer Bacup
3 Bath Place
Rivington Street
London EC2A 3DR

Cancer Link
17 Britannia Street
London WC1X 9JN

Cancer Research Campaign
10 Cambridge Terrace
London NW1 4JL

Continence Foundation
307 Hatton Square
16 Baldwins Gardens
London EC1N 7RJ

Digestive Disorders Foundation
3 St Andrews Place
London NW1 4LB

Family Planning Association
2–12 Pentonville Road
London N1 9FP

Hysterectomy Association
Aynsley House
Chester Gardens
Church Gresley
Swadlincote
Derbyshire DE11 9PU

IBS Network
Northern General Hospital
Sheffield
South Yorkshire S5 7AU

Institute for Complementary
Medicine
PO Box 194
London SE16 1QZ

London School of Aromatherapy
PO Box 780
London NW5 1DY

Macmillan Cancer Relief
3 Angel Walk
London W6 9HX

National Endometriosis Society
50 Westminster Palace Gardens
Artillery Row
London SW1P 1RL

National Institute of Medical
Herbalists
56 Longbrook Street
Exeter
Devon EX4 6AH

National Osteoporosis Society
PO Box 10
Radstock
Bath BA3 3YB

Natural Progesterone
Information Service
PO Box 131
Etchingham
Kent TN19 7ZN

Premature Menopause Support
Group
PO Box 392
High Wycombe HP15 7SH

Relate
Herbert Gray College
Little Church Street
Warwickshire CV21 3AP

Women's Health Concern
Wellwood
North Farm Road
Tunbridge Wells
Kent TN2 3DR

Women's Health Concern
PO Box 1629
London W8 6AU

Women's Nutritional Advisory
Service
PO Box 268
Lewes
East Sussex BN7 2QN

INDEX